Making Medical Choices

Making Medical Choices

Who Is Responsible?

JANE J. STEIN

With a Preface by David A. Hamburg, M.D.

HOUGHTON MIFFLIN COMPANY
Boston 1978

Library of Congress Cataloging in Publication Data

Stein, Jane.
  Making medical choices.

  Bibliography: p.
  Includes index.
  1. Medical ethics. 2. Medicine—Decision making.
3. Medical innovations—Moral and religious aspects.
I. Title. [DNLM: 1. Ethics, Medical. 2. Delivery
of health care—United States. 3. Technology, Medical.
W50.3 S819m]
R724.S83   174′.2   78–14226
ISBN 0–395–27086–3

Printed in the United States of America

v 10 9 8 7 6 5 4 3 2 1

To Bob, with love

Acknowledgments

THE DRAMAS of medical decision-making described in this book are acted out daily. The circumstances of each case differ, but the underlying question — what kind of life do we want for ourselves and our family? — remains constant. No one person can answer this question, but many — philosophers, physicians, health-policy planners, and each one of us, healthy or sick — contribute to its resolution. I sought answers from them all.

In the two years in which I researched and wrote this book, I interviewed nearly two hundred persons who are concerned with the morals of medical decision-making. I owe special thanks to LeRoy Walters and James Childress, of the Kennedy Institute for the Study of Human Reproduction and Bioethics, in Washington, D.C., and to Daniel Callahan and Robert Veatch, of the Institute of Society, Ethics and the Life Sciences (The Hastings Center), in Hastings-on-Hudson, New York. The personal attention and encouragement they gave me, plus the liberal use of their libraries, were crucial for my research efforts.

At the Georgetown University Hospital, Dr. Mary Kate Davitt, chief of the neonatal intensive care unit, spent much time with me, explaining the technological advances that are so common in our hospitals today, as well as some of the problems they create. At the Spina Bifida Service, Dr. David McCullough and nurse Catherine Quinn carefully reviewed the problems and rewards of treating spina bifida youngsters, and the criteria for not treating them. Nurses Mary McGonagle and Kathleen Foster, at a breast cancer detection center, discussed the inherent conflicts and fears of women seeking mammographies. Dr. John MacDonald, Dr. Charles Tartaglia, and social worker Mila Tecala talked about treatments — both medical and psychological — for terminally ill patients, and Dr. Peter Petrucci and nurse Alise Green invited me to join them on home-care visits, which involve treating dying cancer patients with compassion, not medicines. I thank them all.

I thank, too, Dr. John Berryman, of the George Washington University Medical Center, for the time he spent discussing with me problems of infertility and prenatal treatments, Drs. David Davis and William Knaus for tours of the hospital's radiological procedures and discussions about the controversial CAT scanner, and Dr. Glenn Geelhoed, a surgeon, and nurse Mary Brady, of the intensive care unit, for explaining some of the difficult encounters they have had using life-saving technologies on dying patients.

I am grateful that Dr. Peter Berkman, chief of renal disease, at the Washington Hospital Center, ushered me around the Dialysis Center. Dr. James Collins reviewed some of the psychiatric aspects of treating patients with end-stage renal disease, and Dr. Charles Currier, a surgeon, talked about the promises of renal transplantation as a way to treat chronic kidney failure.

I also thank the many other physicians in Washington with whom I spoke: internists and cardiology specialists Drs. Michael J. Halberstam and Joseph Romeo talked about the confusion surrounding coronary artery bypass. Dr. Richard Edelson, a neurologist; Dr. Jay Grodin, a fertility specialist; Dr. Frank MacMurray, an internist; and Dr. Robert Murray, a geneticist, all spent time discussing with me the ethical impacts of their specialty areas. I am grateful to the numerous researchers at the National Institutes of Health for insights into the problems and promises of their work. Among these researchers are Drs. Roscoe Brady and Carl Merrill, both of whom are working on advances that may ultimately lead to treatments for genetic diseases, and Dr. Malcolm Martin, who is involved in recombinant DNA research. Fred Bergmann, director of the genetics program at the National Institute of General Medical Sciences; Dr. Nancy Cummings, associate director for Kidney, Urologic, and Blood Diseases Programs at the Institute of Arthritis, Metabolism, and Digestive Diseases; and Nancy Wexler, executive director of the Commission for the Control of Huntington's Disease and Its Consequences, also offered much information and insight. And I thank Dr. Philippe V. Cardon, associate director of the Clinical Center; John Fletcher, adviser on ethics to the director of the Clinical Center; and Charles McCarthy, chief of legislation, for their contributions on ethics issues.

Many other medical centers were hospitable to me during the course of my research, and I should like to give my special thanks to the following New Yorkers: Dr. Christopher Bryan-Brown, director of the Falk Surgical-Respiratory Intensive Care Unit at Mount Sinai Hospital; at the Albert Einstein College of Medicine, Dr. Bertrand Bell, professor of community medicine; Dr. Harry Gordon, director emeritus of the Rose F. Kennedy Center for Research in Mental Retardation and Human Development; and my brother-in-law, Dr. H. David Stein, assistant professor of surgery. Also, Sidney Rosoff, president of the Society for the Right to Die. In New Haven, Dr. Raymond Duff, of the neonatal intensive care unit at Yale–New Haven Hospital; the Reverend David Duncombe, chaplain of the medical school; Angela Holder, medicolegal adviser to the hospital; hematologist Peter McPhedran; and surgeon Bernard Siegel were especially helpful.

Several members of the University of Connecticut Health Center were of great assistance. Dr. Robert Greenstein, geneticist and chairman of the Committee on Human Experimentation; Joseph Sheehan, chairman of the Department of Medical Education and Research; Dr. John Raye, chief neonatologist; and Stuart Specker, philosopher and associate professor of community medicine, shared their insights with me. In Boston, Dr. Melvin Levine, director of Ethics Rounds at Children's Hospital, and Dr. Mitchell Rabkin, medical director of Beth Israel Hospital, reviewed ethically laden medical policies at their hospitals. And in Denver, Dr. Albert Haverkamp graciously spent time discussing the developments of, and the controversies about, fetal monitoring.

Health-policy analysts also contributed much to this book, and I should like to give special thanks to the following: Dr. H. David Banta, at the National Center for Health Services Research of the Department of Health, Education, and Welfare, for his views on medical technology; Dr. John Bailar III, editor of the *Journal of the National Cancer Institute*, for his comments on mammography; William Blanpied, director of the Office of Ethical and Human Value Implications of Science and Society at the National Science Foundation, for introducing me to the conflicts of technology and health care; and Richard Rettig, at the RAND Corporation in Washington, for his analysis of the federal government's kidney disease program. Allan Fox, legislative assistant to Senator Jacob Javits; Harold Green, director of the Law, Science, and Technology Program at George Washington University; and Stanley Jones and Michael Pollard, both of the Institute of Medicine, all helped provide a better understanding of legislative aspects of health-care policy and the growing movement toward public participation in scientific and medical decisions.

At the National Commission for the Protection of Human Subjects of Biomedical and Behavioral Research, Albert Jonsen, commissioner and associate professor of bioethics at the University of California (San Francisco) School of Medicine, answered many questions thoughtfully, and Barbara Mishkin and Betsy Singer assisted in providing me with reams of appropriate documents. Members of the Maryland Commission on Hereditary Disorders were also helpful in giving me information. Special thanks go to former chairman Shepherdson Abell; Dr. Neil Holtzman, a member of the commission; and administrative assistant Marian Robertson. Public health nurse Sue Crosby and nutritionist Elizabeth Walker, who faithfully attend the commission's monthly meetings, talked at great length about the problems of detecting and treating youngsters with phenylketonuria (PKU).

These are some of the people who helped provide background information, which was so necessary for the development of this book. But the real sources of information were the scores of individuals who wrestled with ways to resolve medical decisions for themselves or for someone in their family. All the cases related in this book are true; they are based on information given me by patients, family members, and physicians, and on documented medical accounts in the professional journals. Some people preferred to remain anonymous, and, in these cases, I took the liberty of assigning them fictitious names. They, however, know who they are, and I thank them silently. To the many people who willingly gave up their time as well as personal privacy to discuss these crucial issues with me, I give special thanks: Ann and Shoshanna Abeles, Marylou and Nick Barr, Bill and Sally Brown, Beverly and Rose Marie Carter, Phyllis Holton, Nancy Karl, Kay Katz, Gay Kroeger, Annie Oliphant, Gay Polyzois, Lorraine Schuler, Carolyn Sinclair, George Terry, Kay and Michael Teague, and Jocelyn Wilks. Without their stories, the book could not have been written.

I am especially indebted to Dr. H. David Banta, James Childress, Dr. Robert Greenstein, Dr. H. David Stein, and LeRoy Walters for reviewing the manuscript, and to Dr. David A. Hamburg for writing the preface. Charlotte Andrews deserves a commendation for her rapid typing of the final version; Daphne Abeel, my editor at Houghton Mifflin, is appreciated for her encouraging words; and David Wise proved himself a valuable friend by urging me to write this book and providing helpful suggestions once I began it. My husband, Bob, and children, Stephanie and Jeremy, are especially thanked for their endearing patience and love while I worked, seemingly incessantly — long days and weekends — in researching and writing this book.

For everyone who helped me write this book, for everyone apprised of the issues who reads it — indeed, for everyone — I hope it will be a helpful guide through the difficult medical choices that will inevitably arise during a lifetime.

Preface

THE CENTRAL THEME of this book is that technological advances in medicine have created a multitude of choices for each individual — choices that can influence how we live and die. These choices are difficult ones, and the book provides a better understanding of the issues. Thus, the implications of each choice become clearer. Such decisions remain inherently very difficult and personal. We need to think hard about these choices, which in some ways are unprecedented. We need to learn more about ways in which individuals cope with such problems, the useful processes of decision-making, and the social conditions that foster effective resolution of conflict.

Making Medical Choices deals with complex and poignant dilemmas. Under what conditions, or burdens, should children be brought into this world? Screening for genetic diseases can help prevent birth defects, yet there are ethical problems — from coercion to social stigma — as exemplified by experiences with PKU, sickle cell, Tay-Sachs, and Huntington's Disease.

The quality of life can be directly related to the delivery of health care. In neonatal intensive care units, lives are saved as premature babies as small as two pounds continue growing outside the womb but in womblike environments. Yet attempts are made to save all babies — including fetuses of brain-dead mothers and babies with no visible hope of a meaningful life. Who has the right to make the painful decision of which baby lives, which baby dies? Should our vast but ultimately limited medical resources be used on everyone regardless of condition — every deformed baby, or every person with end-stage renal disease? The government's decision to pay for virtually everyone who wants dialysis is a landmark in decisions that will have to be faced about the expenses and responsibilities of health care. Today, one hears more than ever before about advances in biomedical science and technology on the one hand and about constraints on health care resources on the other. How can these be reconciled? In the long run, will the former help to solve the latter?

Thoughtful, compassionate societies must consider these difficult problems. Can we develop mechanisms to assist in the medical choices that will inevitably take place throughout each individual's life? Jane Stein makes a stimulating effort to clarify these subjects in this book. She calls to attention problems we would prefer to avoid, touches the untouchable, and in so doing contributes to a constructive debate on the future of human life.

David A. Hamburg, M.D.
President
Institute of Medicine
Washington, D.C.
April 1978

Contents

Making Medical Choices

Chapter 1

Medical Mores

Most people care about their health only when it is too late — when they lose it. This loss of good health can now be controlled by medical technology, from the moment of conception to impending death. But the ability to control life is an awesome tool, and it opens a floodgate of ethical conflicts that are unavoidable and sometimes insoluble.

The myth of anyone's being immune to these conflicts is fading, as more and more men, women, and children — through personal actions, environmental conditions, and genetic predispositions — are made sick and are forced to face the dilemmas caused by medical advances. The truth is that no one is immune. From life through death, medical technology intrudes into our lives, as it did in the lives of the following four people.

Several medically related decisions — each one carrying with it important ethical implications — faced Marian Carter, a thirty-eight-year-old mother of two children, when she became pregnant for the third time. Should she have another child? If she did, she wanted it to be normal and healthy, like her other two children. Should she take a test that would tell her whether or not she would have a mongoloid baby, one with Down's syndrome? The chance of a mother younger than thirty having a mongoloid is only one in 2000, but the risks increase sharply with the mother's age. One mother in every 100 between the ages of thirty-five and thirty-nine bears a Down's child, and for mothers between the ages of forty and forty-four the risks are one in fifty.

Amniocentesis held the clue. In amniocentesis, a small amount of amniotic fluid is removed from the uterus by a needle inserted into a pregnant woman's abdomen. This fluid contains fetal cells, which can be examined for abnormalities of development. Down's syndrome is caused by a chromosomal abnormality, and it is easy for the doctor to detect such an abnormality by analyzing the fetal chromosomes shed into the amniotic fluid. What is more difficult is the mother's decision either to have an abortion or to bring a mongoloid child into the world — if the test discloses abnormal chromosomes.

For Marian Carter, having an amniocentesis involved making a value judgment about what kind of child she wanted: normal or retarded. She had the amniocentesis, and the laboratory tests showed normal chromosomes. Her third child was born just like her other two — normal.

⟨When Gail Kalmowitz was born two months prematurely on May 5, 1953, she weighed a perilously low two and a half pounds. As was standard treatment in those days, she was put in an incubator that was infused with high concentrations of oxygen. Physicians were in a tight ethical bind. They knew that many of the small premature babies saved from certain death with the incubators became blind, but the cause of the blindness was not known. Was it related to the incubator lights? A vitamin A deficiency? Answers were only speculations.

It soon became apparent that high levels of oxygen caused the blindness, but this medical information came too late for Gail Kalmowitz, who had her right eye removed when she was six and has limited left-eye vision. (She reads Braille and is now a psychologist, training to work with blind children.) Without the oxygen therapy, however, Gail would have very likely died or been so oxygen-starved that she would have had permanent and serious neurological damage.

If Gail were born today at the same weight, she would be

placed in a neonatal intensive care unit and plugged into a vast array of life-saving apparatuses. Although all of these seem safe, one new machine or drug used today may ultimately be harmful, the way high oxygen concentrations are now known to be harmful. Knowing the alternatives — death or severe handicaps — should doctors or parents deny babies life-saving techniques because of possible harm? Does the risk of a new medical procedure outweigh the benefits?

￼John Chambers, a foreign service officer in the U.S. State Department, began suffering chest pains when he was in his early forties. Within a few years, he was diagnosed as having severe coronary disease. He had to limit some of his activities, including jogging — one of his favorite forms of exercise. A surgeon friend told him about the wonders of coronary artery bypass, a new procedure designed to reduce chest pain caused by clogged coronary arteries, the conduits that supply the heart muscle with the oxygen it needs to pump effectively.

Chambers questioned a cardiologist at the State Department about the procedure and was told that "bypass" is costly (a typical operation costs between $10,000 and $15,000), carries a 10 percent mortality risk, and is not warranted in all heart conditions.

Further diagnostic tests, in which Chambers's arteries were viewed by means of an arteriogram, confirmed the cardiologist's belief that bypass was not a recommended procedure for this patient. Chambers, however, sought a second opinion from his surgeon friend, who recommended surgery — though he could not give Chambers a promise of a cure, relief from pain, or an extended life.

Whom should Chambers have believed? What assurances should he have got in exchange for a 10 percent risk of dying from an operation?

He sided with the cautious cardiologist, who put Chambers on a gradual exercise program. Now, six years later, Chambers jogs three miles daily, has a normal cardiogram, and is flying around the world on State Department assignments, as he was before his chest pains grounded him. Yet if John Chambers had had the surgery six years before, he would no doubt attribute his renewed state of good health to the operation.

❲Sloan Oliphant was sixty-five years old when he died, two years after he was diagnosed as having cancer of the esophagus. He had surgery, during which several inches were cut from his intestines, but the surgery was purely a stopgap measure, to alleviate pain; his cancer had already spread to other parts of his body. He kept losing weight and became weaker and weaker. Radiation treatments were prescribed by his physician, but, according to Oliphant's widow, Annie, "My husband would be so weak when he came home from the treatments that he couldn't even make it up the front walk to the house."

Halfway through the treatment program, Sloan and Annie Oliphant knew two things about the radiation series: they weren't going to make Sloan any better, and they gave him great discomfort. The Oliphants made the decision jointly to stop the technological interventions that were postponing the time of Sloan's inevitable death.

Technological Highs: Interventions and Expectations

From diagnosis to cure — or to palliative measures that prolong the life of the dying — how we are born, live, and die depends more and more on medical technological advances. The benefit-risk equations of these advances are unknown: they may prolong life as much as shorten it; they may increase the quality of life as much as decrease it. What is irrefutable is that the Pandora's box of medical technology is open.

Medical technology is still a relatively young field. Fifty years ago, the term "technology" would have been out of place in a discussion of medical practice. Physicians identified diseases, predicted their outcome, and guided the patient and the family while the illness ran its full, natural course.

Measures were taken to relieve pain, but most of the measures were of unproven effectiveness. Genuine therapeutic remedies were rare — vitamin C for scurvy, quinine for malaria, morphine for pain, digitalis for heart failure — and surgery was restricted largely to emergency measures, such as removing or draining areas of infection, repairing broken bones, and removing a few types of cancer.

In half a century's time, biomedical practice has changed its approach from using what Dr. Lewis Thomas, author of *Lives of a Cell*, calls nontechnologies to halfway technologies, a change from diagnosing and reassuring the sick to using technological interventions that compensate for, but do not cure, certain diseases. Transplantations of kidneys, hearts, and livers are all heroic measures taken after a disease has caused irreversible damage.

The causes of the two leading medical killers, heart disease and cancer, are poorly understood, and much of today's therapy for managing them relies on halfway technologies. Sophisticated electronic devices for monitoring patients in coronary care units, specialized ambulances for transporting coronary patients, battery-powered cardiac pacemakers, and coronary artery bypasses are measures for dealing with the end results of heart disease. And the only possible course for treating cancer is to destroy the affected tissue by surgery, radiation, or chemotherapy. Nothing can reverse the damage caused by these diseases.

High technology, in contrast, aims directly at the underlying causes of diseases, to stop, reverse, or, best of all, prevent them. The conquest of polio epidemics is a good example of a successful high technology. A simple and inexpensive vaccine replaced the complex and expensive halfway technology of iron lungs and artificial limbs. Immunization has, with both efficiency and low cost, eliminated or vastly reduced numerous other devastating diseases within a few generations. Smallpox, measles, diphtheria, whooping cough, tetanus, rabies, yellow fever, and many more are controlled through immunizations. But this technology is not without problems, as public health specialists wrestle with vaccine-caused deaths and illnesses, liability, compensation, and the conflict of voluntary versus mandatory immunization programs.

Tuberculosis treatment, too, moved from its halfway technology state, in which the progressive destruction of lung tissue was "treated" with mountain spas, sunlight, prolonged rest, and surgery. In the early 1950s, just before the introduction of a high technology to treat TB — antibiotics — there was an elaborate nationwide plan to install facilities for thoracic surgery in TB hospitals. The costly building program for a halfway measure was replaced by a relatively inexpensive and very efficient drug. A vaccine, when it is developed, will be the ultimate high technology for protection against tuberculosis.

Antibiotics, which also deal effectively with pneumonia, syphilis, meningitis, and other bacterial diseases, are still not a perfect technology because some growths are resistant to them. This problem is increasing — not lessening — because antibiotics are used, and often overused, for common minor complications, making once treatable bacterial strains immune to the drugs. In addition, new strains of such serious diseases as pneumonia and gonorrhea are appearing on the list of infectious ailments resistant to antibiotics.

The list of high technologies goes on: injection of insulin in diabetics whose natural supply is missing or limited, prevention of Rh disease in newborns by injecting anti-Rh antibodies in mothers (in contrast to the risky removal and replacement of the infant's total blood supply). But it is a short list, and there are not nearly as many "cures" as the public is led to believe.

Ironically, the complex halfway technologies are enticing and keep people in awe of medical advances. TV viewers watched an amniocentesis procedure live on the "Today" show, and Shep Glazer, a New Yorker with kidney failure, demonstrated before the House Ways and Means Committee in Washington how his dialysis machine cleanses his blood of bodily wastes, a function normally done by kidneys. Glazer's performance helped get federal financial coverage for victims of terminal kidney disease.

The public remains attracted to devices that have an increased capacity for controlling life, and expectations of the benefits of these advances are high. In a survey of 600 families, commissioned by Chicago's Mount Sinai Hospital Medical Center, one third of those questioned thought that 60 percent of lung cancer patients survive, although only 10 percent in fact do. "The public thinks we can fix anything now," said Dr. Leroy P. Levitt, the hospital's vice president for medical affairs.

But "the public's expectations from medical technology are somewhere east of Mars," said Dr. Bertrand Bell, professor of community medicine at the Albert Einstein College of Medicine in the Bronx, New York. "The uses of technology are limited because they affect very small numbers of people. We are not going to cure cardiac diseases with coronary artery bypass operations. The body's pipes are rusty, and what is needed are new pipes, not diversions around the rusty ones. The whole technology of cardiac surgery is ridiculous, but it is an example of the public's expectations of technology."

Because science can treat — or is expected to treat — a wide variety of diseases, health care has become a bigger and more significant consumer of society's resources. New treatments are being invented faster than they can be assessed or even paid for. As the total annual volume of resources devoted to health grows — $150 billion were spent in 1977, but $250 billion will be spent each year in the 1980s — there is a sharper awareness of resource constraints and the need to make choices.

Yet more, not fewer, medical tools are sought, and the public clamors for more, not less, money to be spent on health. In a survey sponsored by the National Science Foundation, more than two thirds of those responding listed "improving health care" as the area on which they most wanted to have science and technology tax monies spent.

Although the public generally places medical technology on a high pedestal and secretly hopes to wake up to read in the morning headlines that a cure for cancer has been discovered, there is a growing movement against relying on technology, and a damnation of the medical profession for playing God. We can create, prolong, and terminate life. But should we?

Several recent events stimulated the public to question the medical technological fix. In the 1960s, the Thalidomide tragedy — in which thousands of children were born with gross physical defects, and uncounted fetuses mercifully died — pointed out the need for better monitoring of drugs and highlighted the problems of exposing humans, however unknowingly, to detrimental yet effective therapies. Thalidomide, after all, was an excellent sedative.

When artificial kidney machines changed from being used as temporary life supports for acute cases of kidney failure to long-term supports for chronic kidney disease, three disturbing questions were aired publicly: What kind of meaningful life can a person have if he or she is dependent on a machine? Who will decide which patients are worthy of using the scarce and expensive dialyzer? Who will pay for this expensive medical therapy?

Another development that provoked ethical examination was the success of transplantation. The need to get donors for hearts, kidneys, and livers forced the issue of redefining death and using brain death as a medical criterion, so that the healthy organ can be removed as soon as "death" occurs and before organ deterioration begins.

As other extraordinary means of health care began to proliferate — respirators, artificial parts, and surgical techniques to save or prolong lives of the very sick who would die without radical treatment — the question was raised more acutely:

Should we be using all the medical technology we have developed?

Fear of genetic manipulation because of laboratory advances in recombinant DNA research was the final factor in catapulting the issue of medical ethics into public consciousness. With the ability to control genetic make-up by using recombinant DNA techniques — combining genes of different species and inserting the newly formed genetic material into foreign cells — came the ability not only to control health and fitness, but also to reconstruct the human species.

Ethical Principles, in Codes and in Practice

Interest in medical ethics is not new. Since the time of Hippocrates in the fourth century B.C., there have been medical codes, guidelines, and prayers. What is new, however, is the change in emphasis: Hippocrates was concerned more with the medical etiquette of the physician's relationships with his patients and fellow physicians than with the morality inherent in medical decisions.

The Oath of Hippocrates serves as a contractual agreement between the novice physician and teacher, as well as a set of restrictions on medical techniques used by physicians. According to the oath, physicians promise to do no harm, and in keeping this promise they may refuse to grant certain requests, such as pleas for poisons and abortive remedies. (These standards sharply contrasted with actual Greek medical practice, which permitted physicians to encourage suicide and infanticide.) The oath also defines the physician's relations with the patient's family; he or she promises to provide confidentiality, not to commit acts of injustice, and to abstain from having sexual relations with women, slaves, and men in the household.

The first great modern code was *Medical Ethics: Or, A Code of Institutes and Precepts Adapted to the Professional*

Conduct of Physicians and Surgeons, published in 1803 by Thomas Percival, an eminent physician in Manchester, England. Percival advised physicians to treat patients with compassion, fidelity, and humanity, to consider benevolence and virtue more than wealth and rank in determining fees, and to avoid use of fraudulently advertised medicines. He also urged physicians to keep their heads clear and hands steady by observing strict temperance.

When the American Medical Association was organized in 1847, it adopted a Code of Ethics drawn largely from Percival's. The AMA's code wanted to set standards for medical practice in hopes of re-establishing public respect for the medical profession. In the mid-nineteenth century, numerous quacks, lacking orthodox training, posed as medical practitioners; they used secret remedies, patent medicines, and claimed to have "special" abilities to cure.

Over the years, the AMA ethics code updated Percival's ethics for running a medical practice. It is still unethical to use a secret remedy on a patient, but abortions are no longer unethical, when done in accordance "with good medical practice and under circumstances that do not violate the law." The bulk of the AMA code, however, covers the ethics of running a modern medical practice, including fee-splitting, charging for missed appointments, and complying with insurance company requests for information about patients.

The scientific and medical advances of recent years have raised ethical questions of a more life-and-death nature in a number of areas not covered by the AMA code. As a result of the growing success and popularity of organ transplants, the AMA issued guidelines on the ethics of transplantation, cautioning the physician to protect the rights of both the donor and the recipient. And development of techniques to keep a dying person alive indefinitely raised ethical and legal questions about the responsibility of attending physicians. AMA guidelines for treating the terminally ill were developed, authorizing the physician to abide by decisions of the patient or the immediate family to discontinue extraordinary efforts to prolong life when evidence of imminent death is irrefutable. (Guidelines for recognizing this irrefutable evidence, however, were not provided.)

In 1972, the American Hospital Association adopted a Patient's Bill of Rights, changing many of the rules of medical practice, which for more than 2000 years stressed the physician's dominance. According to the bill, the physician is no longer the sole authority in managing the patient or deciding what information to give. Decision-making about a course of treatment is now shared with the patient, a right that, in theory, the patient always had but rarely asserted. While the Patient's Bill of Rights applies only to patients in hospitals, it sets a precedent that physicians may eventually be obligated to follow.

*

Codes have moved slowly from etiquette ethics to what is now called bioethics: the study of the moral and social implications of practices and developments in medicine and the life sciences. Even the definition of health has moral and social implications. "Health," according to the definition adopted by the UN's health agency, the World Health Organization, "is a state of complete physical, mental, and social well-being and not merely the absence of disease or infirmity." This is an ambitious definition, giving medicine an enormous mandate. No wonder the public has such high expectations from medicine.

"With minor ingenuity, anyone can make a desire seem a health need," commented Daniel Callahan, director of the Hastings Center, an ethics think-tank in Hastings-on-Hudson, New York, "and any health need can be legitimated in the name of the right to health. The political system cannot make all of the people happy all of the time, but it is just possible that physician-prescribed psychotropic drugs can." Is happiness a health requirement — or a value?

Why not remove, as a prophylactic measure all the breast tissue of baby girls at birth, a procedure that would cost but a fraction of the money invested in the care and treatment of breast cancer and on research for its cause and cure?

Because it is "a question of values," answered physician-philosopher H. Tristram Engelhardt, Jr., professor of the philosophy of medicine at the Kennedy Institute for the Study of Reproduction and Bioethics, Georgetown University. "Deciding what counts as health requires a decision about what counts as an appropriate goal for man . . . These are philosophical problems as much as they are medical problems."

Consider the notion of rights. Is there a right for a person to be born with a healthy genetic constitution, to have access to his or her medical records, for physicians to practice where and how they please? What are the limits of rights? In some states, a fifteen-year-old girl can have an abortion without her parents' consent, but she needs their approval to have an appendectomy.

Consider also the principle of autonomy, or self-determination. Can a sick person be an autonomous person? Being sick means being in an abnormal state. A sick person may be more anxious than a healthy one, or may have faulty perceptions. If patients are not autonomous, who should be responsible for their actions? Are physicians responsible to their patients or to society? A precedent for their being responsible to society already exists: physicians are required to report confidential patient information about contagious diseases to public health officials.

*

Medical decisions — many with philosophical implications — are often demanded of us throughout life. Should Marian Carter have had an abortion if the prenatal diagnostic test showed that her fetus was a mongoloid? Should Gail Kalmowitz's family have refused to let the physicians place her in an oxygen-infused incubator? Should John Chambers have chosen to have the coronary artery bypass? Should Sloan Oliphant have tried a few more months of radiation treatment in exchange for a few more months of life? Each of these medical decisions involved ethical values. Treatment has become a question of values.

The issue of giving informed consent for medical procedures provides a good illustration of the ethical problems in medicine. There is no procedure or drug that does not have some possible adverse reaction. Any surgery could be followed by pulmonary embolism and death. Even common aspirin may cause suffocation. If patients give their informed consent for a certain procedure or drug, does this consent protect them from harm? Does it give them enough information on which to make a rational decision? Or does it protect the providers — the physician and the hospital — from liability?

Radiologists at the Cleveland Clinic studied more than 200 patient reactions to general disclosures of possible complications resulting from an angiogram, a diagnostic procedure for studying blood vessels. The consent form explained that the artery would be punctured under local anesthesia and that there would be a small possibility of clotting, which would then require surgery to remove the clot, and a remote but nonetheless real risk of loss of an organ or of life. The dye used in the procedure might cause hives, low blood pressure, or, in rare cases, temporary or permanent paralysis. The consent form added that the rate of serious complication following an angiogram is one out of 500.

All scary stuff, and though as many as one-third said this information made them uncomfortable, only four patients out of 232 refused the angiogram after receiving the information. It is rare for a person to refuse to have an appendectomy, when it is medically justified, because of the fears aroused by a consent form, but the Cleveland researchers point out that the angiogram is a diagnostic procedure, not a therapeutic one.

How beneficial to the patient is all this information? Researchers at Montefiore Hospital in the Bronx reported that no matter how carefully patients were briefed before consenting to open-heart surgery — they were told about the surgery, devices that would be used, benefits, risks, potential complications, and alternative methods of therapy — postoperative interviews showed that they failed to remember most of the information. Some patients even denied any recollection of the preoperative interview.

Is it ethical to ask patients to sign a consent form they will probably forget? Is it ethical to do a procedure without obtaining their permission? In an emergency situation, informed consent is usually waived before treatment begins. Would it be ethical to let a man lie unconscious in the emergency room, waiting for him to wake up so that he can give the doctor permission to perform life-saving surgery?

Each situation is different from another, and in medicine there is no one absolute answer to ethical questions; there are, instead, many. The increasing reliance on medical technology complicates the matter. Before much of the life-sustaining technology existed, there was no problem in deciding when a patient should be taken off a respirator. There was no respirator. And there was no way of evaluating the quality of life of a person on triweekly dialysis treatments. There were no dialysis machines. With new developments in medical technology, dilemmas are constantly created where none existed previously.

Caution is needed in dealing with these constantly developing bioethics dilemmas, and an ethics backlash has already developed. The new concern with ethics is viewed as representing antiscience or antitechnology feelings, and ethicists are castigated by some members of the scientific community for focusing more on the harm that may be done to individuals than on the hazards to the general public that may result from the inhibition of scientific advances.

Some people think that ethics means finding something bad. But to flag a problem as one of ethics is not to blame or condemn, but, rather, to alert the public to inherent dangers so that action can be taken to avoid or lessen them. The subsequent chapters of this book will flag many ethical issues that are commonplace in the practice of medicine as it spans a lifetime — from before birth, through life, and on to death. Although they are commonplace, most of these issues are not yet commonly perceived as ethical concerns.

I

BIRTH

Chapter 2

Creating a New Life

A BABY IS BORN, a miniature person who developed perfectly during the nine-month period from the moment of conception to birth. In awe, proud parents think, "Isn't the creation of life so beautiful, so simple?"

For more and more parents, the answer to this question is *no*. The very creation of life can now be manipulated and enhanced through various kinds of medical intervention. Couples previously infertile are having babies, thanks to drugs, surgery, and artificial insemination. And couples who have had children with severe mental and physical handicaps because of genetic mistakes can have each subsequent pregnancy tested, give birth to the normal babies, and abort the defective ones.

Most of the advances to control the beginning of life have been developed within the relatively recent medical past. It was not until 1956 that the correct number of chromosomes in humans — forty-six in every cell except for sperm and eggs, each of which has twenty-three — was properly identified. Chromosomes, which contain all the genetic information that is needed for growth, can give researchers clues about the development and potential of each human being.

Too many or too few chromosomes usually indicate trouble. A person born with an extra Number 21 chromosome in all or many of the cells will be a mongoloid. An extra Number 13 chromosome usually results in a mentally retarded child, with a small, malformed head and with an extra finger on each hand. The defects of infants born with too few chromosomes are usually so incompatible with life that the babies die soon after birth, if not before.

There are also defects in the thousands of genes that make up each chromosome. The blueprint, or set of instructions, for producing a person is written in these genes in a genetic code, which is actually chemical compounds arranged in a building block. A small mistake in the code alters the building block and can prevent the formation of a protein or enzyme essential to healthy growth and development.

Genetic errors do not always mean disaster, and it is believed that minor genetic defects are very common, occurring in 6 to 14 percent of all live births. These defects — birthmarks, flat feet, premature white hair, color blindness, myopia — are not considered serious medical problems.

But there are more than 3000 genetic diseases that result in mental retardation, crippling physical deformities, and other defects that compromise a child's development to a full and normal life. Five percent of the children born each year are victims of these genetic mishaps. The severity of genetic diseases is highlighted by the following statistics:

❧Forty percent of all infant deaths are due to genetic factors, and more than one third of all spontaneous abortions are caused by gross chromosomal defects.

❧Infants who survive a major genetic defect are virtually assured a life of illness. One third of the children admitted to hospital pediatric wards are there for genetic-related reasons.

❧These tragedies are not as rare as the public thinks. Each of us carries five to eight genes for serious genetic defects, and each married couple has a 3 percent risk of having a genetically defective child.

Because of the increased ability to create and control life — as well as the trend toward curbing population growth — parents are beginning to assert themselves: "If we have only two children, let them be free from genetic defects."

In the Beginning

Scientific advances can create life but cannot give us an exact answer to the question of when that life is created. Philosophers today are no nearer to agreement on when life begins than were the Greeks. Plato believed that life begins at birth, but Aristotle disagreed with his master and held that the male has a soul, or life, forty days after conception. Females, according to the Aristotelian scheme, develop their souls after eighty days. Early Islamic theology placed the beginning of life at a different point in time: life was thought to begin 180 days after conception.

When does life begin? Does it begin at the moment of conception, when the egg is fertilized by the sperm? When this union takes place, there is present all the genetic information that the new individual inherits organically. The hereditary potentialities in that fertilized egg then begin to unfold: three weeks later the heart beats, six weeks later the fetus moves, and by twelve weeks it is sucking its thumb, swallowing, digesting, and urinating. These early fetal responses are only quantitatively — not qualitatively — different from early to late pregnancy, according to the proponents of the life-begins-at-conception thesis.

Or does life begin when the fertilized egg becomes implanted in the wall of the uterus, usually a week after fertilization? The egg has already divided repetitively and has become a ball of cells, or a blastocyst. When it becomes implanted, it causes a signal for the mother to switch her reproductive functions from a nonpregnant to a pregnant condition and to create a new human being in the uterine environment.

Yet another theory proclaims that human or personal life begins when the fetal brain begins to function. The soul is frequently associated with the mind, and until the brain is functioning there can be no mind. Starting in the seventh month of pregnancy, electric potential from brain waves is detectable when electrodes are placed on the mother's ab-

domen over the fetus's head. Are brain waves a valid sign of
life, just as the absence of brain waves is a valid sign of death?

*

All the evidence points to a lack of scientific proof as to
when life begins. There is no definable moment of conception, implantation, or the first wave of brain activity. Human
life is, instead, a continuum, and fertilization, implantation,
and the first brain wave are merely three events in its unending cycle.

In recent years, the issue of defining life has changed from a
debate about the point at which it begins to one about the
point at which it is possible outside of the womb.

The court decision of the celebrated Edelin case of the
mid-1970s, in which Kenneth Edelin, a Boston obstetrician,
was first convicted and later acquitted of manslaughter in the
death of a legally aborted fetus, did not even try to resolve
the issue of when life begins. But it did rest part of its case
on the American College of Obstetricians and Gynecologists'
definition of a live-born infant: "a fetus, irrespective of its
gestational age, that after complete expulsion or extraction
from the mother, shows evidence of life — that is, heartbeats
or respirations."

A fetus is viable when it is capable of becoming a live-born
infant — when it can live independently from its mother.
This state is usually reached during the last three months of
pregnancy. Until then, the fetus is dependent on the mother
for full realization of its potential — for nutrition, oxygen,
waste removal, even for its own metabolism. But with technology's help, fetuses as small as one pound are surviving outside the womb. Is this, by definition, a viable life — or is it
more a statement about technology's ability to keep hearts
and lungs functioning?

By whatever definition is used, medical technology can
control the creation of life, from the very union of sperm and
egg to the quality of that union. The power that parents, the
medical profession, and society have over the formation of

new human beings is staggering. Is the immensity of this responsibility a blessing or a curse?

Making Babies

There is a sizable minority — 15 percent of all married couples — who need help in getting the basics of life, sperm and egg, together. The classic question of which comes first, the chicken or the egg, is painfully illustrated for infertile couples: without the egg's being released — the process of ovulation — there can be no baby. But there is a simple course of treatment in which ovulation can be induced in 98 percent of the cases: a drug can stimulate the follicles of the ovaries, inducing them to release the eggs they hold. Normally, this job is done by female hormones.

Getting an egg to drop can be risky. A hormone-releasing drug that is commonly used results in a 25 percent chance of multiple births, from twins to sextuplets. Women taking the drug often develop ovarian cysts, which are removed surgically, but occasionally the ovaries burst from overstimulation, with lethal results.

There are other maneuvers that can enhance the joining of egg and sperm. Plastic reconstructive surgery unblocks fallopian tubes, the passageways through which unfertilized eggs travel to meet the sperm. And uteruses that are not strong enough to support a growing fetus for nine months are shored up with surgical supports.

The problem is not exclusively that of the female. In about 40 percent of the cases of infertility, the male is either wholly or partly sterile or his sperm is not motile enough to cause pregnancy. About half of the men who have some sperm are made fertile by hormones that stimulate sperm production or by surgical repair of sperm-inhibiting varicose veins in the testicles.

"All these operations and drugs, and the promise of more," said Dr. Jay Grodin, a Washington, D.C., fertility specialist who has helped thousands of couples to have children, "yet we cannot give any couple the assurance that these techniques will result in their having a baby."

There are still a large number of couples who cannot be helped by modern treatment. Adoption was formerly a realistic option for them, but since abortion became legal, safe, and readily available, adoptable children have become scarce.

Infertile couples, therefore, in ever-increasing numbers, choose to get sperm and egg together through physical manipulation: by having the gynecologist insert sperm from a donor directly into the woman, in the hope that it will fertilize a waiting egg. Each year an estimated 10,000 to 20,000 children are born by artificial insemination by donor (AID). So successful is this procedure that 95 percent of the parents come back for a second child, and 37 percent request a third. Less commonly performed is artificial insemination by husband (AIH), when the husband has sperm but is unable to transport it effectively to his spouse, usually because of such physical handicaps as paralysis or obesity.

In spite of the fact that about half a million Americans have been conceived by artificial insemination, only a few states consider their births legitimate. Most were born into, and live their lives in, legal limbo.

Adultery and illegitimacy are the principal issues clouding the legality of artificial insemination. Is a child entitled to support by the mother's husband? Can the doctor be accused of conspiring in the commission of adultery? Because of these legal questions — even though the majority of recent court decisions hold that the artificially inseminated child is legitimate — most physicians recommend that the husband and wife sign documents consenting to the procedure, agreeing to raise any resulting child as their own.

Artificial insemination poses many uncertainties in addition to the legal ones. Theoretically, one donor could produce enough semen to create 20,000 babies a year, raising the issue of lack of random selection. What is being sought, however, is not an assembly-line production of children, but a way out of infertility. Although there is a possibility that AID children conceived from the same donor could marry and have children, it is very unlikely indeed. Nevertheless, most physicians limit the number of live births for which each donor contributes sperm.

Another often-raised issue concerns truth-telling: Are AID children told of their true parentage? Virtually every physician doing artificial insemination recommends that the child *not* be told about the procedure. It would raise anxieties unnecessarily, they argue, about who the real father is, but since there is no way to trace the sperm back to the donor, there is no identifiable father. One woman who was told of her donor parent — a rare disclosure — recalled that "knowing about my AID origin did nothing to alter my feelings for my family. Instead, I felt grateful for the trouble they had taken to give me life."

In most cases the paternity is intentionally clouded. When a husband produces some sperm — no matter how few or how weak — they are mixed with the donor's sperm. Sometimes couples are urged to have intercourse after the insemination to add to the doubt and to increase the sense of the husband's participation.

"The only thing a man gives up in artificial insemination by donor is that he substitutes someone else's genes for his. The rest is the same — going through nine months of pregnancy with his wife, and the birth of the baby," commented Dr. Grodin.

Artificial insemination explodes some questions about the ethics of medical practice. "Fertility specialists are placed by their patients in a God-like position," said Dr. John Berryman, director of the fertility clinic at the George Washington University Medical Center in Washington, D.C. "We are asked to help parents get the babies they want but can't have. Couples become so desperate, they seek help from quacks and charlatan sex counselors, falling prey to anyone who promises to help them, just as people flock to diet doctors who charge three hundred dollars for vitamin shots."

Consider the cases of three couples, each of which spent five years trying artificial insemination. In all three cases the woman's fallopian tubes were closed. "There was no way those women could get pregnant," Berryman said angrily. "Yet they spent a hundred and fifty dollars a month — ninety dollars for the donor semen and sixty dollars for the office visit — in their futile efforts."

Or consider another couple in search of having a baby. The wife didn't ovulate, and the husband was misdiagnosed as having inadequate sperm. They went for artificial insemination treatments for eighteen months, for an insemination that wasn't warranted and in a woman in whom it couldn't work.

Medical technology can get eggs to drop and sperm to flow. It can implant sperm and now, after more than two decades of futile attempts, can attach a fertilized egg to a woman's uterus.

In 1959, Daniele Petrucci, an Italian scientist, announced to the press that, after more than forty attempts, he had fertilized a human egg *in vitro*, in a test tube, and sustained the embryo alive in this artificial environment for twenty-nine days. At that point he terminated his experiment, because the embryo "had become deformed and enlarged, a monstrosity." If that fertilized egg had been reimplanted in a woman, grown to full size, and delivered, who would have been responsible for the "monstrosity": Petrucci or the parents?

"It is one thing to accept for yourself the risk of a dangerous procedure if the purpose is therapeutic . . . It is quite a different thing deliberately to submit a child, born or unborn, to hazardous procedures which can in no way be considered therapeutic for him," wrote physician-philosopher Leon Kass in the *New England Journal of Medicine*.

In the mid-1970s, human egg and sperm, fertilized in a test tube, were reimplanted in a woman four days later by two British physicians, Drs. Robert Edwards and Patrick Steptoe. They reported in *Lancet*, a British medical magazine, that the fetus died after ten weeks because the pregnancy developed in a fallopian tube rather than in the womb itself. The two

British physicians were not discouraged, and after scores of unsuccessful embryo transfers, the first baby conceived outside of a mother's womb was born in 1978 — a healthy girl at birth. The baby's mother had been unable to become pregnant in the normal fashion because her fallopian tubes were irreversibly blocked.

Meanwhile, government-funded research on test-tube fertilization in the United States was halted in 1975 until the ethical issues surrounding it could be cleared up. But the National Ethics Advisory Board, which was to review these research requests, was not even appointed until three years later.

Implantation of a fertilized egg raises questions about the limits and function of medicine. Providing a child by artificial means to a woman with blocked fallopian tubes is not a treatment, as surgical reconstruction would be. The woman remains as infertile as before. What is being treated is her desire to bear a child.

Are doctors playing God or simply trying to help infertile couples to have children? Would only infertile women use this procedure, or would wombs be hired by women who want to have children but wish to avoid pregnancy and childbirth for the sake of their careers, convenience, fear, or vanity?

There may be some prospective hirers, but most women would not elect to use the surrogate-womb route to motherhood — unless they could not reproduce because they lacked eggs or their fallopian tubes were blocked.

"The issue is not wombs for hire," said Dr. Cecil Jacobson, a Washington fertility specialist who had pioneered in test-tube–baby research in this country. "The issue is an infringement of freedom of rights — people telling you that you can't have a baby. The ban on egg-transfer work is sexism on a genetic level. Why can we use male semen and not female eggs for procreating outside the body?"

*

Hiring a womb has already happened.

"Childless husband with infertile wife wants test-tube baby," read a want ad in the San Francisco *Chronicle*. The childless husband was the last of his family line, and he wanted a child — his own child — to carry on the family name. He chose artificial insemination because, he said, "it would be immoral to have a sexual relationship outside of marriage to father a child." He said that his wife had been somewhat doubtful about the idea at first, but then had agreed to go along with this approach to parenthood.

He never met the mother of his child — chosen from among more than 180 respondents — but she was described as "an attractive, blond, unmarried office worker living in the San Francisco Bay Area" who had never had a child before. She rented her womb for $7000, and produced a five-pound, six-ounce red-haired girl. Said the proud father's lawyer, "It is exactly equivalent to artificial insemination of women by anonymous donors."

The ever-fertile mind is compensating for infertile bodies. Creating babies can be done. Should it be forbidden, or used wisely, carefully, and as a last resort for bearing healthy, normal children?

Everyone Doesn't Have Normal Children

Kay and Barry Katz live in the suburbs with their two young children. Bikes are parked in the garage, and two cars are in the driveway. They look like a typical young family, but it is only because of advances in medical technology that they dared to have "the family we got married to have," said Kay, a former schoolteacher.

The Katzes were at first denied this family because of genetic defects that they unknowingly passed on to their first-born child, Joann, who died a pitiful death before she was four years old. Joann was a victim of Tay-Sachs disease, a cruel condition in which the central nervous system degenerates. Tay-Sachs children look normal at birth, but within a few months motor weakness begins, and gradually they can no longer crawl or sit up. Eventually there is paralysis, blindness, convulsions — all due to a progressive buildup of a fatty material in the central nervous system. The fat deposits, called lipids, are normally broken down by an enzyme that Joann and other Tay-Sachs children lack.

Tay-Sachs disease is a classic recessive disorder in which each parent carries a normal gene for the functioning of the enzyme, hexosaminidase A, and a recessive harmful gene for its absence. Each child from that union has a 25 percent chance of being normal — getting the normal genes from both parents; a 25 percent chance of being affected — getting the defective genes from each parent; and a 50 percent chance of being just like each parent — carrying a normal and a recessive gene.

Tay-Sachs is a rare disease for most people. But Jews of central and eastern European ancestry have a high incidence of it. One Jewish birth in every 3600 will be a Tay-Sachs baby, in contrast to one baby in every 360,000 among non-Jews.

Kay first heard about the disease when she was pregnant and read an article about it in a magazine. "I became alarmed," she recalled as she talked in her kitchen a few days before Joann would have been seven, "but many alarming things happened during my pregnancy. My grandmother died of cancer, and two months later my mother had a mastectomy. I began to bleed and had to spend a week in bed. I remember thinking: here I am lying in bed when I should be teaching. And for what — to avert a miscarriage? Maybe I should just let nature take its course."

Kay was upset enough about what she had read to discuss it with her obstetrician, who tried to reassure her that Tay-Sachs was a very rare disease. "I was seven months pregnant at the time, and all the advice he could give me was to worry or not to worry. There was nothing he could do." In retrospect, Kay feels that it was irresponsible of her physician not to suggest that she see a genetic counselor.

The Katzes' anxieties were relieved when Joann was born, two months later — eight pounds, healthy, and beautiful.

But within a few months, Kay began to sense that there was something different about her daughter. "Other babies seemed more vigorous and robust, but she lay like dead weight in my arms. I was frightened, but I couldn't express it. I tried rationalizing that every baby develops differently and that she would outgrow it. I tried every excuse."

By eight months, Joann sat up, talked — but never rolled over, never made an attempt to crawl, clap her hands, put things in her mouth, or transfer toys from one hand to another.

At nine months, she began to wake up screaming.

And by ten months, the decline set in. She couldn't sit up by herself anymore. "Just the month before, she sat up on the pediatrician's scale, and now she had to lie down on it," Kay remembered. "When I pointed this out to the doctor, he said, 'Don't worry. My daughter didn't sit up until she was thirteen months old. This is all perfectly normal.' "

"But," sputtered Kay all those years later, "his daughter hadn't been able to sit before. She was progressing while Joann was declining. Why didn't he see the difference?"

When Joann was eleven months old, the pediatrician admitted that she was not developing normally, and she went to the hospital for a series of tests on her bones, blood, thyroid, muscles, and brain.

"We brought Joann home from the hospital the day before her first birthday with the knowledge that she had Tay-Sachs disease, that the birthday cake placed in front of her the next day would be the only one she would ever see, and that she would no doubt be dead before her fourth birthday," said Kay, remembering that sad day.

And that was exactly what happened. Joann died at three and a half, a blind invalid, suffering seizures and drowning in her own secretions, requiring daily enemas, surviving on a liquid diet fed through a tube plunged down her nose into her stomach.

"These were the real events we had to stand by and helplessly witness, and when you love someone the way we loved Joann, you would do anything to reverse the insidious process that was taking her away from you, and, short of that, anything to prevent its recurrence."

Kay and Barry wanted to have children but would not risk having another one with Tay-Sachs. And they knew that they had a 25 percent chance of having a Tay-Sachs child with each pregnancy. They also knew it was possible to detect the presence of Tay-Sachs prenatally by amniocentesis, the same procedure that had allowed Marian Carter to know that the fetus she was carrying did not have Down's syndrome.

"We had a big decision to make because we desperately wanted more children of our own," Kay said. "After several months of soul-searching, we agreed to go ahead and plan a second pregnancy. Seeing Joann deteriorate convinced me to go ahead with the amniocentesis and have an abortion if Tay-Sachs was detected. Although the idea of an abortion wasn't a very pleasant one, it was better than bringing another Tay-Sachs baby into the world."

The odds were favorable for Kay and Barry, and the next two pregnancies resulted in two normal children.

"Now we have a family because prenatal diagnosis and the option of abortion allowed us to become a family, even though I never needed to have an abortion," reported Kay.

*

For the Katzes, as for most couples, the birth of a defective child came as a surprise. They knew nothing about their genetic history and the risks they faced with each pregnancy. But with hindsight — knowing the risks as well as knowing that something could be done about them — the Katzes avoided a second tragedy.

"These days you have a choice about having a healthy baby," said a young woman who had had a Tay-Sachs child and was pregnant again and waiting for the results of an amniocentesis. Although this statement is not exactly true —

the next pregnancy could result in a child free of the genetic defect but with an unrelated heart problem — it reveals a willingness to rely on medical technology.

There are additional ways of detecting genetic conditions prenatally. By viewing the fetus indirectly by means of a sonogram (a computerized picture made by sound waves), the physician may note gross physical defects, like a very large or very small head, either of which is often associated with severe mental retardation, dwarfism, and spinal defects.

The fetus can also be viewed directly by use of a fetoscope, inserted into the amniotic fluid. This long, skinny needle has a tiny optical device at the tip equipped with lenses and a light. There is also room in the 1.7-millimeter-diameter fetoscope for a second needle, by which fetal blood samples can be drawn from the placenta and analyzed to determine if the fetus has sickle cell anemia or other inherited blood problems. Fetoscopy is a far riskier procedure than amniocentesis, but it allows the doctor to do more. With amniocentesis, the physician can neither draw fetal blood samples nor detect sickle cell disease.

Spina bifida, a major cause of birth defects, can be diagnosed prenatally by a study of the mother, not the fetus. Traces of a fetal protein that leaks out from the fetus into the pregnant woman's blood or urine are telltale signs of this physically crippling and mentally retarding condition.

Though amniocentesis is the most reliable and widely used of the prenatal-detection procedures, it is still relatively scarce, mostly limited to university-associated hospitals in major cities. The few thousand women who have the procedure done yearly are a self-selected, well-off group. A study of nine major U.S. medical centers found that more than 90 percent of the women having amniocentesis are white, half are college-educated, and most have above-average incomes.

"I know I can get a diagnosis to see if I'm carrying a normal child and terminate the pregnancy if I'm not," Kay Katz said. "But it isn't right that a poor black woman of forty-five, with five children and pregnant with the sixth, doesn't even know

— and is rarely told — about a test to see if she is carrying a mongoloid child."

Risks, Rough Times, and Rationalizations

The insertion of a needle into a woman's uterus carries with it the theoretical risks of maternal infection, spontaneous abortion, or injury to the fetus. Studies, however, consistently show that there is virtually no difference in the percentage of fetal deaths among pregnant women who have had or have not had amniocentesis. Nor is there a greater chance of adverse complications during or after pregnancy for the mother or child, except when more than one needle insertion is made to get the fluid; these complications can often be avoided if sound waves are used to locate the placenta and the exact position of the fetus.

Accuracy of diagnosis is a source of greater concern. The accuracy rate is 99.3 percent, which sounds very high except if you are one of the unfortunate few on whom the error is made.

A survey of 1040 pregnant women who had amniocentesis showed an incidence of six errors. Two involved children born with Down's syndrome, both of whom had been diagnosed as not having the abnormal chromosome make-up of mongoloids.

There were three errors in sex determination, but these had no medical consequences since the diseases being looked for were not sex-linked (as is hemophilia), and one infant was normal but had been wrongly identified as having a metabolic disorder, galactosemia (an inability to metabolize milk), which may result in severe mental retardation. The parents had decided not to abort the fetus, because the condition is treatable if the baby is given a strict diet that includes no milk.

The timing of amniocentesis poses potential ethical problems. Most experts recommend that the test be done no earlier than the sixteenth week of pregnancy. Before then, there is a chance that the amount of amniotic fluid will not be sufficient to cushion and protect the fetus from the needle. Also, before sixteen weeks, the fetus often has not shed enough cells into the fluid to supply the information that is being sought.

It takes an average of three weeks to analyze the fluid and to develop cell cultures from it. This means that if Kay Katz had been given a positive diagnosis that she carried a Tay-Sachs fetus, she could not have had an abortion until close to the twentieth week of pregnancy. What further complicates the problem is that the fetal cells do not always grow in the culture, and occasionally another sample must be taken, adding three more weeks to the waiting period.

Abortions done between the twentieth and the twenty-fourth weeks of gestation not only present more frequent and serious physical complications for women than do earlier-term abortions; they also approach the borderline period for viability. It is almost inevitable that a positive diagnosis of a genetic disease and a subsequent late abortion of the fetus will result in a live birth.

*

The roughest time for most couples is waiting for the report on amniocentesis ("We shouted at each other and fought like tigers," recalled one husband), but when the report shows a defect, things become even rougher. Many couples become very depressed — and with good cause.

These women and men are seeking normality, not an abortion. They grieve the loss of their normal child, feel guilty about having conceived a defective one, and are afraid that they will do so again. Women who are repeaters — those who have had previous abortions for genetic reasons — bear vivid memories of their disappointment and sense of failure.

Psychological problems can be avoided, insisted Dr. Jacobson, who counsels couples in his fertility clinic. "The best way to take care of the situation is to advise the couple that they will be under stress until they follow that pregnancy with the birth of a normal child." Consider the case of a woman who had had an abortion after the prenatal test confirmed that her fetus was affected with the same rare disease that her first child had. "My marriage was rocky for at least eight months after the abortion," she admitted, "and it took two years — until the birth of our normal son — to become completely stable."

*

A stillborn birth can be considered an act of God, but an abortion requires a human decision. Many couples rationalize that it is their parental and social responsibility to have an abortion because of genetic defects. The major arguments in favor of this decision are based on the obligation to reduce suffering and to prevent genetic disease for future generations.

"It's not fair to the child, to the family, to society, or to me to bring into the world another child like the one I have," said the mother of a child with a rare disease that results in severe mental retardation, palsy, and bizarre desires for self-mutilation. She was diagnosed as carrying another son with this disease, Lesch-Nyhan syndrome, and had an abortion.

Or consider the forty-two-year-old mother who said, "I have two children and did not intend to get pregnant again. But I did, and now I must do everything possible to see that my child is healthy. I would have an abortion if it were defective. The world has enough problems, and I don't want to add to them."

Most couples at risk for bearing a child with a genetic disease do not regret having the prenatal diagnosis. Those who get good news are greatly relieved by the knowledge that their child will not have a dreaded handicap.

And despite the emotional trauma suffered by those couples who receive bad news, most indicate that they will have the diagnostic test again and will selectively abort any future pregnancy if the test indicates a defective fetus. They agree that this route, with all its problems, is preferable to the alternative: the birth of a defective child. "After seeing what our first baby went through, there was nothing to think about in deciding to have an abortion," reported a mother of a Lesch-Nyhan son. "It is hard to feel guilty after seeing that baby suffer." These families have known the depression that abortion can produce, but they also know the tragedy of genetic illness.

Although the option to abort an affected fetus is an underlying assumption in the parents' decision to have an analysis of the amniotic fluid and the fetal cells it contains, abortion for genetic reasons is surprisingly rare — as the Katzes discovered. Among the women who underwent the diagnostic test because they suspected a birth defect, 97 percent were reassured that the defect in question was not present.

Prenatal diagnosis assumes abortion as an option, but it is called a life-saving procedure because it makes childbearing possible for people like Kay and Barry Katz, who might otherwise be afraid to have babies. Barry Katz once responded angrily to an anti-abortion group that was exhibiting pictures of aborted fetuses. "I've seen your pictures. Now do you want to see mine? Here's a picture of my daughter who died of Tay-Sachs, and here's a picture of my two children who are alive and well. They wouldn't be here if we couldn't have had amniocentesis and detection, and the option to abort. Don't take away our rights to have a family; don't prevent the birth of healthy, normal children."

The Ambiguities of Prenatal Detection

Francine and John Giordano both come from large Italian Catholic families in New England. They were still arguing about how many children they would like to have when Elizabeth, their first child, was born. And that almost put a stop to any considerations of a normal family. Elizabeth was born with a rare disease, recognizable at birth, that results in severe mental retardation and grotesque physical features. This condition, unlike Tay-Sachs, is not a life-threatening one, and

Elizabeth could live her severely compromised life for decades, well into adulthood.

The Giordanos faced their responsibilities for their daughter — all the medical, social, economic, educational, and psychological problems that were involved. Even though they loved Elizabeth dearly, defects and all, they wanted to have a normal child and a normal family life.

When she was pregnant again, Francine had an amniocentesis, and the laboratory tests showed that she was carrying a fetus with an unusual chromosomal make-up: parts of two chromosomes had broken off and exchanged positions. In genetics, this is called a translocation. In a balanced translocation, chromosomal pieces exchange places without losing any material. But in unbalanced translocations, some genetic material is lost, usually resulting in serious birth defects.

What did this translocation mean: normal or abnormal development? The Giordanos could not be told, with accuracy, anything about the chromosomal aberration. Most people described as having translocations are in mental institutions, but that does not mean that all people with translocations are mentally retarded, because it is not known how many of them are in the normal population.

In Francine's nineteenth week of pregnancy, she and John sought out other prenatal diagnostic measures. Fetal head circumference can be measured by means of a sonograph. If the head is of normal size, then there is an indication — though not a 100 percent assurance — that development is progressing normally. But if the head size is very small, it may be an indication of abnormal development.

The Giordanos' luck was waning; the sonogram reading indicated a small head size. At the same time, Francine's obstetrician felt that the uterus was smaller than it had been in a previous checkup, further indicating but not assuring abnormal development.

The Giordanos had already made the decision for Francine to have an abortion, based on their fear of having another abnormal baby. They had reached their decision with great sadness. But that decision was soon questioned. In a routine check on Francine before the abortion, a second sonogram revealed normal fetal head size.

Which report was correct? Francine could no longer take the lack of definite information, and she went ahead with the abortion. An autopsy was performed, and there was neither fetal malformation nor small head size. But the meaning of the translocation was still unanswered.

The Giordanos adopted a normal baby girl. Elizabeth, now four, is very retarded, and it is likely that she will never learn even to sit up by herself. And then there is Maria, the Giordanos' normal two-year-old. Should they have taken the chance, continued with the second pregnancy, and risked the possibility of having another abnormal child? Who has the right to answer this question? The medical profession? The policy makers at hospitals where abortions are performed? Or the Giordanos, and thousands of couples like them, who want to choose the kind of family life they hope to have for themselves and their children?

With medical technological advances come some of the tools to help the Giordanos and others make this difficult decision. But as this story shows, sometimes the tools give misleading or inconclusive information, and the decision-making process becomes even more difficult.

*

The science of prenatal detection is far from perfect: only 100 out of more than 3000 genetic conditions can be determined with accuracy *in utero*. And even some of these diagnoses are ambiguous.

Consider the options of prenatal detection available to victims of Gaucher's disease, an enzyme deficiency that in one form attacks the central nervous system and may result in severe mental retardation and death in early childhood. Not all youngsters are as severely affected, and those who have even a little of the missing enzyme — as little as 20 percent of normal production levels — have full intellectual capabilities and can lead relatively normal lives, except for periods of severe pain and burning sensations in their hands and feet due to nerve damage. "We can diagnose Gaucher's disease prenatally and we can tell parents if there is less than ten percent of the normal enzyme activity — a condition that leads to severe mental retardation — or if the fetus is producing twenty percent of the normal enzyme production, in which case nerve-ending pain is the biggest problem," said Dr. Roscoe O. Brady, an expert in Gaucher's and other enzyme-deficiency diseases, working at the National Institutes of Health. "But we are not clear about the outcome of those with enzyme activity hovering between ten and twenty percent. I think they are not likely to have mental retardation. But this is not yet a scientifically proven fact. What should the parents do: abort or continue the pregnancy?"

Brady has no answers. "I don't tell anyone what to do," he said. "But I do tell them what will happen — when I know it."

Ambiguity in prenatal decision-making is perhaps the greatest in diseases that cannot yet be diagnosed from amniotic fluid but are manifested only in one sex. Sex can be easily determined through chromosomal analysis of fetal cells. The gene for hemophilia, a blood-clotting deficiency, is carried on one female sex (X) gene, and there is a 50 percent chance that each male child conceived by a carrier will have the condition. Parents then have the option of aborting all male fetuses to avoid having one child with the disease.

Carolyn Sinclair found herself in an unusual and ambiguous genetic situation. Her first child was mentally retarded, had stunted growth, and abnormalities in his heart and lungs. He was diagnosed as suffering from one of two diseases, Hurler or Hunter syndromes, which are similar clinically and biochemically but have different genetic roots. Hurler's is a recessive genetic disorder carried by both parents (as is Tay-Sachs), but Hunter's is a sex-linked disease, carried only by the mother and passed on only to males (as is hemophilia). Carolyn's first husband, Jeff's father, had died in an automobile accident, so if Jeff had Hurler's, which is caused by a double dose of genes, she had no worries about this happening again (unless she had the unlikely misfortune of marrying another man with a recessive gene for Hurler's syndrome).

But Jeff was diagnosed as having Hunter's, and Carolyn's physician told her that if she married again and wanted children, there would be a 50 percent chance of her having another son like Jeff. Carolyn soon after married Charles Sinclair and became pregnant. "I had always wanted to have four sons," recalled Carolyn, "but now I prayed for a daughter."

Carolyn's luck wasn't with her, and the amniocentesis she had indicated that she was carrying a boy. At that time, medical researchers had not perfected methods of determining the biochemical differences between affected and normal Hunter cells, so the Sinclairs had to decide whether to accept a 50 percent risk of having another abnormal son or to have Carolyn undergo a therapeutic abortion. They decided on the abortion rather than face the possibility of raising two retarded children. "We couldn't afford to have another child like Jeff — financially or emotionally. It's more emotionally draining than I could ever explain," Carolyn said.

The next decision the Sinclairs faced was whether Carolyn should become pregnant again and perhaps go through the whole ordeal, including an abortion. Should they adopt? Should they not have any more children?

While the Sinclairs were pondering these questions, Carolyn became pregnant, had another amniocentesis, and got the bad news again: another boy. Once more she had a 50 percent chance of having an abnormal child. But in the year and a half since her first amniocentesis, medical researchers had been busy decoding more mysteries from the amniotic fluid, and they could now precisely determine from the fetal cells the presence or absence of Hunter's disease. "This is an enormous responsibility," said Dr. Elizabeth Neufeld, the biochemist at the National Institutes of Health who analyzed

Carolyn's fetal cells, "predicting what a life will be like, based on a biochemical test."

There was more waiting while the cells grew and were analyzed, but luck finally prevailed for Carolyn, and the male child she carried was free of the disease that had stunted Jeff's size as well as human potential. "I do not plan to have any more children," Carolyn said. "I do not want to go through this again. With two sons — Chris, who is normal, and Jeff —I've been very lucky." Carolyn was not as lucky with her marriage. The stress of caring for a sickly and retarded child places an enormous strain on normal family life, and the Sinclairs were subsequently divorced.

*

As the chemical clues to more and more genetic diseases become unraveled, some of the chanciness and ambiguity of genetic counseling will be alleviated, as it was, finally, for the Sinclairs. "As the diagnostic net gets larger it will, unavoidably, catch conditions other than those for which it was intended." This is the fear expressed by Dr. Neil Holtzman, a pediatrician and geneticist at the Johns Hopkins University School of Medicine and a commissioner of the Maryland Commission for Genetic Disorders. "What is to be done if a condition is discovered in the fetus that is of unknown consequences or only mildly debilitating or effectively treatable?"

Are there any limits to prenatal diagnosis? Few parents of children with Tay-Sachs would disagree about abortion for a fetus with Tay-Sachs disease. Think of Kay, Barry, and Joann Katz. Life after the birth of a second Tay-Sachs child would have been devastating for the parents. There is less agreement about abortion for mongoloids. Troublesome issues lie in wait, as more and more conditions are detected prior to birth, as more and more control is gained over life.

Chapter 3

Manipulating the Gene Pool

SCREENING FOR a genetic disease is like looking for a needle in the haystack: it is a search for those in the population who have such a disease or carry the means to pass it on to the next generation. The stakes are high, and the prize is the prevention of birth defects.

Medical technology has advanced to the stage where it is possible for scientists to conduct large-scale searches for dozens of genetic conditions in the hope of reducing the frequency of a disease, and helping families at risk to learn more about the disease and ways to prevent or treat it. The goals of screening are noble-sounding, but they are not without problems. The most troubling aspects of genetic screening and of learning more about each person's genetic make-up, in fact, are not scientific or technological but ethical. As new information unlocks many of the mysteries of genetic diseases, it forces the making of decisions that may ultimately alter the gene pool.

Reaching the Masses

An inexpensive and painless test — analyzing blood taken from a pinprick on a newborn's heel, or urine sopped up from a wet diaper — can determine within a week or two after birth whether or not that infant is a victim of phenylketonuria (PKU), an inborn error of protein metabolism that leads to severe mental retardation if it is not properly treated. Unlike some other genetic conditions, PKU cannot be detected before birth, nor can parents be identified as carriers of it. But once a PKU child is born, the parents soon know that they are carriers and that each subsequent pregnancy carries a 25 percent risk of ending up as a PKU baby.

PKU children cannot properly use a substance in protein, the amino acid phenylalanine, and it begins to pile up, spilling over into the blood stream and urine, where it can be detected. This buildup damages the baby's fast-growing brain, although researchers are still not precisely sure how this damage occurs. Five to 6 percent of the proteins found in normally available food are made up of phenylalanine, so if foods containing a larger proportion of protein — breads, milk, meat, cheese — are kept out of the diet, brain development will not be significantly impaired. The only natural foods not containing phenylalanine are sugar and vegetable fat.

The benefits of screening for PKU are clear, according to Dr. Holtzman, who helped to draw up Maryland's PKU screening procedures. "PKU youngsters score five points lower in IQ tests than their brothers or sisters and may not perform quite up to par with other children. They may have behavior and learning problems, and they may not go to the best college, or to any college. But they are within normal limits. Untreated PKU children, those who are not screened, form quite a contrast. They are severely retarded children."

Screening for PKU makes such good sense, even though it affects only one in 14,000 births, that most of the states followed the example of Massachusetts, which passed legislation in 1962 requiring that all newborn children be tested for PKU. Some of that legislation is now being reviewed and repealed, as problems with the testing procedure and ethical issues related to it have emerged.

The heralded test is not foolproof. Some infants are identified as false positives — as having the condition when they do not. Researchers have discovered that not all children with elevated phenylalanine levels have PKU. There is a range of metabolic disorders, hyperphenylalaninemias, not all of which justify the protein-restricted diet that PKU children need, a diet that can be harmful to normal growth because phenylalanine is essential to brain development.

Conversely, there are a significant number of PKU babies — 10 percent — slipping by the screening net. They are either not being screened or are identified as false negatives — that is, they are assumed not to have the disease when they do.

An infant screened in the first three days of life is more likely to be missed than a six-day-old infant because of quirks in the progression of the disease. It takes time for the baby to drink enough milk so that the phenylalanine in it builds up and flows over to the blood and urine, making it easily detectable. Furthermore, levels rise earlier in males than in females, so baby girls with PKU who are screened during the first few days are at an even higher risk of being missed. "Screening during the first four days of life is not sensitive enough," Holtzman pointed out, "but it is the least costly program, because infants can be screened before they are discharged from the hospital."

An alternative way to test babies over three days old is to have the mother put a specially treated paper on the baby's urine-soaked diaper during the infant's second or third week of life, and mail it to health authorities. This is not a foolproof method, either: not all parents are diligent about doing the test, and public health officials are lax about following up those who do not comply.

The need to identify PKU babies early in life is essential, because the earlier treatment begins, the better the outcome. Infants who begin following the proper diet within the first three weeks of life have a better outcome than those who begin it at six weeks.

In this instance, all that stands between the right to good health and mental retardation is an inexpensive, easy-to-do blood or urine test. Whose right is this? The child's to receive? The parent's or the state's to provide? Should the test be mandatory? Voluntary?

Mandatory screening has an odious aspect to it; it could well be a prelude to an enforced policy of eugenics, to weed out what the state decides is an undesirable genetic characteristic. A panel of experts convened by the National Academy of Sciences emphatically opposed mandatory screening and came out with strong recommendations to have existing PKU legislation modified and to make all screening voluntary.

The reasoning is based on sound ethical principles, but *not* requiring the test also has profound ethical implications. After Maryland made PKU testing a voluntary procedure, the state's Commission on Hereditary Disorders began receiving reports that 250 of the state's 50,000 babies born each year do not have the test because their mothers refuse to give permission for it. Although this is a very small percentage of births — 0.5 percent — it still affects a sizable number of babies. What will happen when a PKU baby not detected at birth reaches the age of two? Will the parents realize that their child is irreversibly retarded because they refused to have the test done? Will they blame the state because the test was voluntary, not mandatory?

What happens to some people when PKU testing is voluntary and haphazardly run can be devastating. Consider the predicament of Ann Maguire, the mother of three PKU children, one of whom is so profoundly retarded that he has been institutionalized for more than a dozen years. The annual cost of institutional care in Pennsylvania, where the Maguires live, is $20,000 per child and is rising each year. In comparison, screening for PKU costs less than $1.00 per child.

Ann Maguire's first two children, John and Billy, were born with PKU, undiagnosed and undetected until the damage was permanent. Then the Maguires had three normal children. In 1967, when Christine was born, she looked perfectly normal, but she soon began to show some of the signs that her older brothers had shown — weak motor movements and a strange urine smell. But she was tested for PKU, and, her mother reported, "I was of the impression that the test had exonerated Christine from the disease." Christine had slipped through the net, and, though it was undetected at birth, her PKU condition is very apparent today. Although not as profoundly retarded as Billy, she does have to go to a special school for mentally retarded children. Mrs. Maguire feels that "appropriate treatment at the appropriate time would . . . have left my children normal children in every respect."

The biggest problem of having children with PKU, according to Ann Maguire, "is that they all could have been well because of the diet." Knowing all of this, she added, "It is really not easy to have to visit your child at a state institution, either."

Ann Maguire testified in Washington before a congressional committee on how health policies are shortchanging children. She said that the only way to prevent "this horrifying disease" is by having a mandatory, effective detection program, with no one going undetected, no one going untreated.

*

Mandatory screening for sickle cell disease seems to have done more harm than good. Intentions were honorable, but the effort was premature. Medically, there is little to offer for sickle cell disease. There is no effective treatment, as there is for PKU, and prenatal detection, on which parents of Tay-Sachs children can rely, is still done experimentally with fetoscopes.

In sickle cell disease, normal round red blood cells have a distorted sickle, or crescent, shape when their oxygen supply is low. These abnormal cells are short-lived, and this higher rate of red blood cell destruction is in part responsible for the chronic anemia that accompanies the disease. Sickle cell disease affects one black out of 500, but the potential for it is even greater: about 8 percent of American blacks, or two million people, have the sickle cell trait, which means they are carriers of a single faulty gene. If carriers marry, there is a 25 percent chance that each child born will have sickle cell disease.

Ironically, what is now called a defective gene was once a life-saving genetic mutation that helped African forefathers survive. Sickling, in some unknown way, interferes with the invasion by the malaria parasite into human red cells, and over the centuries infants with sickle cells had a better chance of surviving their first attacks of malaria than infants with normal red cells. The infants with sickle cells were the ones to survive, grow, marry, have children, and further spread the sickle cell gene widely through the population. Sickle cell trait was a triumph of genetic adaptation.

And sickle cell anemia is the price paid for this genetic adaptation.

Sickle cell anemia is a painful disorder in which oxygen-starved red blood cells stick together and obstruct blood vessels, leading to destruction of local areas of tissue. The severity of the disease varies. Some victims die without ever knowing they have it, but most have some symptoms — as innocuous as slow weight gain and poor appetite — before their first birthday. The blood vessels in joints become clogged with clumps of sickle cells and cause painful swelling. Bouts of pain caused by this clogging are called "crises." Kidneys are often damaged, and blood in the urine is not uncommon. Resistance to infection is low, and pneumonia is perhaps the most frequent cause of death.

In the late 1960s, rapid, inexpensive, and accurate tests for detecting people with sickle cell anemia as well as those with the sickle cell trait became available, and the new ghetto hustle began. There was a rush to screen all blacks for sickle cell without considering what to tell them, whom to tell, or how to counsel. Both counseling and testing were often conducted by people with little training. Misdiagnoses were frequent and misinformation rampant.

The black community that was pushing the screening — a strange combination that included legislators, physicians, and the Black Panthers — was victimized by the very laws they sought to have enacted for protection. Rights were flagrantly violated as states passed legislation for mandatory preschool and premarital blood tests. Blacks also began to realize that, in the wrong hands, a genetic profile could be dangerously discriminatory. Blacks with the sickle cell trait lost jobs, and many were charged higher rates for life insurance policies because employers and insurance companies confused the trait with the disease. (Only those with the disease have a shortened life span.) Some airlines refused to hire blacks with the trait as pilots, stewards, or stewardesses; and deep-sea diving became off limits for them, because of the unknown risk and the fear that the work might precipitate a sickling crisis.

How realistic were these fears? More than three dozen players in the National Football League are sickle cell carriers, and the trait has not caused any impairment of their physical abilities.

The original mandatory sickle cell screening laws and new ghetto hustle failed. But all this is moot, because federal legislation now provides funds for voluntary screening, counseling, and follow-up care. The lure of federal funds is helping to stimulate revision of some of the well-meaning but poorly written state laws, and screening for sickle cell can now proceed to help — and not stigmatize.

*

"We had a tragedy," said Kay Katz about the birth and short life of her daughter Joann, "but it was limited to one child." To help prevent a similar tragedy from occurring, Kay helps organize genetic screening efforts to alert Jewish couples of childbearing age to see if they are carriers of Tay-Sachs and, if both are carriers, to counsel them about the 25 percent chance they have of each child dying as Joann did.

Since the first mass screening program for Tay-Sachs began in the Baltimore-Washington area in 1971, more than 150,000 men and women in the United States have had blood drawn at voluntary screenings in Jewish community centers in seventy-five cities around the country to determine whether or not they are carriers of the Tay-Sachs gene. As a result of these screenings, Tay-Sachs disease has shown a dramatic decline among the Jewish population, dropping from about forty-five births in 1970 to a negligible few in 1978. The reason for this decline is that when couples at risk are identified in the screening, their pregnancies are monitored by amniocentesis; when Tay-Sachs is identified, they select to abort. It is ironic that most of the new cases of Tay-Sachs are discovered among non-Jewish families who are not included in the screenings since they rarely carry the genes for it.

There is no legislation, no legal mandate, yet the screening program succeeds. What are the factors that motivate people to participate in a Tay-Sachs screening? The major reason for the widespread interest is the nature of the disease itself. It is not treatable, and an early and pathetic death is assured for its victims. The disease is not common, even among Jews (one in 900 Jewish couples is at risk for having a child with Tay-Sachs as compared with one in 90,000 non-Jewish couples), but it is easy to prevent — if carriers are identified.

Dr. Michael M. Kaback is a pediatrician-geneticist who teaches at the University of California, Los Angeles, but previously taught at the Johns Hopkins University Medical School. When he was in Baltimore, he orchestrated the first Tay-Sachs mass screening, and he feels that the key to a successful genetic screening is a voluntary approach. "The moral dangers of legislating human genetic testing far outweigh the potential medical benefits," he said. "As a practical matter, legislation alone cannot solve genetic problems. The public must be educated in order for any program to work, and voluntary learning based on enlightened self-interest is inherently more effective than coerced learning."

The technological part of screening for Tay-Sachs — analyzing blood samples for genetic information — is easy. The difficulty lies with the ethical problem of how to help people use that information to make decisions about what kind of lives they want for themselves and their children.

Two of the couples at risk identified in the Baltimore-Washington screening, for example, were engaged to be married. What did this newly found information do to their plans? Should they break up? Have children anyway? Adopt? After counseling, both couples decided to continue their engagement and get married. But since they wanted to have children, they decided that they would have prenatal tests done with each pregnancy and have an abortion if a Tay-Sachs fetus was detected.

A college student identified as a carrier said that because of her religious beliefs she was against having an abortion. "If I marry another carrier," she said, "I would think of alternative ways to have a family — adoption or artificial insemination. But my choice of husband would not be based on whether or not he is a carrier of Tay-Sachs disease."

Another coed disagreed; she did not want a marriage in which she and her husband were both carriers. A twenty-one-year-old MIT student was told that her fiancé, who had been tested for Tay-Sachs in New York, found that he was a carrier. "We are planning to get married in a few months," she told a geneticist at a screening in Boston, "but if I'm a carrier too, we'll take this as a sign that our marriage is ill-fated, and we won't go ahead with it."

Successful as the Tay-Sachs screening program is, only 10 percent of the targeted population — the couples of child-bearing age — have been tested. In Montreal, 75 percent of the Jewish high school students — the next generation of parents — have already been tested, as the effort to reach more people continues.

Is having this information so early in life helpful or detrimental? Ten percent of the teen-agers who were told they were not carriers said they would not marry a carrier, even though such a marital combination could not possibly result in the couple's having a Tay-Sachs child. And 12 percent of the teen-agers identified as carriers said they would "reconsider" marrying their intended spouses if they too were carriers — which means that this group either did not understand or did not accept prenatal diagnosis and abortion as a means of avoiding the birth of affected infants. "Screening for carriers at a time in life when choice of mate is not imminent and when self-confidence ebbs and flows may cause additional problems," Dr. Holtzman warned.

Yet most of the Jewish teen-agers in Montreal know a lot more about Tay-Sachs than do their parents. They know that the disease is hereditary, that a prenatal diagnosis is possible, and most find an abortion an acceptable way not to have a child with Tay-Sachs. These young people will never have to go through the anguish and tragedy that Kay and Barry Katz did.

*

Three different genetic diseases — PKU, sickle cell, and Tay-Sachs; each has different screening objectives, different solutions. There can be "no omniscient guidelines" for dealing with genetic diseases "because the knowledge about screening, counseling, and treatment is constantly and rapidly evolving," reported the American Academy of Pediatrics' Task Force on Genetic Screening.

Variation is not inherently a bad thing. In fact, adapting screening needs to meet the unique specifications of different diseases makes good sense. For Ann Maguire, mandatory PKU screening would have helped her three children victimized by the disease to lead normal lives. But for the blacks who lost their jobs or were otherwise stigmatized because they were identified as carrying a single gene for sickle cell, mandatory screening hurt more than it helped.

Knowing the Risks

Genetic counseling — advising couples about the statistical odds of a genetic mishap and offering reproductive alternatives, such as prenatal detection, abortion, and adoption — must be an integral part of any screening program.

"Our goal is to get the notion of screening — for Tay-Sachs, sickle cell, or whatever is possible — as a routine part of health care, as a common part of premarital counseling," said Dr. Allen Crocker, a Boston genetic specialist.

But who is to do this counseling? Most general practitioners are neither trained nor even interested in issues of genetics. Moreover, a majority of physicians responding to a National Academy of Sciences survey on genetic screening didn't think it was important to be on the lookout for genetic diseases. Perhaps one reason for this lack of concern is that three fourths of the physicians practicing today did not have the advantage of studying genetics at medical school because the subject matter is too new. Genetics courses were virtually nonexistent until the 1960s.

When John Fletcher, a bioethics adviser at the National Institutes of Health interviewed couples seeking genetic counseling, he found that one fifth of them complained that they had met opposition — sometimes open hostility — from their doctors. One forty-year-old mother of three children was told that her mental health needed attention because she sought amniocentesis to avoid having a mongoloid child for which she was at risk.

Kay Katz recalled with great anger what happened when she notified her obstetrician-gynecologist that Joann had Tay-Sachs. "I thought he would like to know more about the disease and diagnostic possibilities since he had many Jewish patients. He wasn't only not interested; he also called me a murderer."

*

Physicians are not the only ones who turn a deaf ear to the matter of genetic predestination. Sometimes the victims of a disease don't want to know the truth about their genetic fate. Huntington's disease (also known as Huntington's chorea, from the Greek word for "dance," because of the jerky, twisting, uncontrollable movements of the muscles in patients) provides a good example of this ambivalence.

There is a good reason for a lack of curiosity about this disease. The reason is fear.

Fear of Huntington's disease is great. Each person at risk has seen a close family member "go crazy" from it — shaking, grimacing grotesquely, going into a rage, becoming paranoid and delusional, symptoms that ultimately result in fifteen years of emotional and physical suffering before death takes over.

For most, the biggest fear is not death or the uncontrollable movements, or even being harnessed to bed to prevent falling out. The biggest fear is loss of intellectual capacities. "You can live with jerkiness, but you cannot live without your mind," said one thirty-year-old woman whose father recently died of the disease. She still has a recurrent dream that her head is turning into oatmeal.

Every child of an HD victim has a 50 percent chance of inheriting the one dominant gene that causes the disease. What is particularly tragic about Huntington's disease is that the symptoms usually appear after the stricken person is thirty-five. By that time, victims have unwittingly passed on the gene to their children, who must grow up with the terrible knowledge that they too may be doomed.

If a predictive test were available — and one isn't at the moment — then those at risk could be relieved of a great anxiety. They could get married and have children without feeling guilty about passing on the disease. They wouldn't have to worry, every time they bumped into the doorway or dropped a dish, that they had the disease. And they wouldn't have that terrible fear.

In a study of thirty-five men and women at risk for HD, psychologist Nancy Wexler, executive director of a commission set up by Congress to devise a plan for the control of Huntington's disease and its consequences, found that not everyone wanted to know if he or she had the disease. Only two-thirds said — with varying degrees of conviction — that they would take a predictive test. And all acknowledged that they would be terrified to take it.

Is the ambiguity of limbo psychologically easier for people to accept than the certainty that they carry the HD gene and have the dreaded disease? The knowledge of having the disease is clearly a disastrous blow. Not surprisingly, the suicide rate starts to climb as symptoms appear, and it is several hundred times the national average by the time patients are diagnosed as having it.

"If I was told that I'm going to get HD when I'm thirty, do you know what every day would be like?" asked a young woman at risk. "Every day would not be a real life. I just couldn't live like that. Now at least I have a fifty-fifty chance. Now I have optimism. It would be good for science to have a predictive test, but it wouldn't be good for the HD victim."

Nancy Wexler holds a different opinion. She too is at risk for Huntington's disease. Her grandfather had it, and her mother and three uncles are victims. Now she and her older sister — both of them in their thirties — are waiting to see if the symptoms develop or if they have been spared.

"I would want to take a predictive test," she asserted. "The gamble is worth it to me. If the answer is no, I'd get married and have children. I would really like to do that. It would be a giant cloud lifted off my head.

"The stakes are high, but the benefits would be worth it. I know I have a fifty-fifty chance of having the disease, but one minute I think it's one hundred percent yes, one minute it's one hundred percent no. Part of everyday life is preparing for the inevitable — the disease — and if the answer were yes, I could cope with having the disease. But being trapped in limbo makes me live a kind of half-life."

Wexler feels that she has a moral responsibility not to pass on the disease to future generations. There are 20,000 victims of HD in the U.S. today, but the disease could be eliminated in two generations if every person at risk decided not to have children.

Many people at risk are willing to gamble, to continue playing Russian roulette, with a 50 percent chance of winning, 50 percent chance of losing. In Wexler's study, one quarter of the couples had children *after* they learned that they were at risk for the disease.

The folk star Arlo Guthrie is in his early thirties and still doesn't know if he inherited Huntington's disease from his folksinger father, Woody, but Arlo already has three children of his own. Woody died in 1967 in a state hospital, after fifteen years of suffering. Arlo's two older half sisters already have been diagnosed as having the disease.

Researchers are working on predictive tests that could indicate the presence or absence of the disease earlier in life — before symptoms appear, before children are born, before the genes are passed on to the next generation.

Skin biopsies of HD patients show an unusual growth pattern. Certain cells called fibroblasts grow and multiply in tissue culture more densely than do normal cells. Perhaps skin biopsies performed on men and women at risk, even on fetuses, could indicate who has the disease. It is unknown whether the fibroblasts show their abnormal growth patterns only as the symptoms appear, or whether they are genetic markers, present at birth.

Huntington's disease victims show another physiological peculiarity: they are deficient in a chemical transmitter of nerve impulses, gamma-amniobutyric acid (GABA). Autopsies consistently show that HD patients have significantly lower GABA levels in brain tissue. Can GABA levels be used in a predictive fashion, or do they show variation from the norm only as the disease progresses? A drug to mimic GABA action is being tested in animals, to see if it relieves symptoms of Huntington's disease, the way L-dopa relieves the symptoms of Parkinson's disease.

The most controversial predictive test involves L-dopa. When it is given to people at risk for HD, it has induced chorea — the shaking, palsied movements — in more than one third of the group. The shaking ceases when the drug action wears off. However, not one person in a group of people *not* at risk for HD developed choreic movements when the drug was given. Some researchers suggest that those people who show signs of L-dopa–induced chorea will develop HD, and those who do not get the shakes from the L-dopa are free of the disease.

A positive test, however, does not prove that the person has HD, though it does indicate that the central nervous system is different from that of a normal person in its response to a dose of L-dopa. A negative response — no chorea — is less meaningful, since it is possible that a person has the gene for the disease but at the time of the test the subject's central nervous system has not been altered enough from the norm to react to L-dopa. Perhaps six months or six years later, L-dopa would produce the shaking movements in that person.

In spite of this inconclusive evidence, some young people at risk want to believe in the results of the L-dopa test. One married woman in her late twenties "passed" the test — she showed no shaking movements — and now feels morally free to have children. But her high hopes may be false: the test is not accurate, and she could still develop the disease and pass on the defective gene to her children. It could take up to twenty years to find out whether the people who react to L-dopa will develop the disease, and whether those who do not develop the chorea while on L-dopa will be spared.

"Huntington's disease is a microcosm of medical research problems," said Nancy Wexler. "Every advance raises an ethical problem." If predictive tests are developed, will the state have the right to force people to take them? Could a person at risk be forbidden to have children — say, by having a mandatory sterilization — or be forced to abort an HD fetus? Does the right to control infectious diseases like smallpox extend to programs designed to lower the number of persons suffering from rare inherited disorders? Is it even ethical to develop a test that would confirm a dreaded fate but provide no benefits — removing all hope, offering no solace?

Normal Children: The Success Stories of Treating Genetic Diseases

For most genetic diseases there are no cures. At best, there is some variety of halfway technology. Hemophiliacs, for example, receive, all during their lives, transfusions of the blood-clotting factor they cannot manufacture themselves. The defect remains, and the damage done by internal bleeding, particularly in leg joints, often leaves hemophiliacs crippled and in constant pain.

One of the most successful interventions for genetic diseases — successful because it allows its victims to lead full and normal lives — is the low-phenylalanine diet for youngsters with PKU. As successful as this approach is — treated PKU children have normal intelligence, but the untreated victims range from mildly to severely retarded — it is still a palliative treatment, not a cure.

One mother of a PKU girl, now a seventh-grader and "just about as average as you can get," remembers vividly when Amy was diagnosed. "I felt frozen as my pediatrician explained that the routine blood test for PKU was positive. And I can still hear him saying, 'You may have a retarded youngster on your hands.' The idea of keeping Amy on her diet terrified me at first. I knew how vitally important it was, and I was afraid I wasn't going to be able to keep to the diet strictly enough. What if I failed? This was my daughter's mentality with which I was tinkering."

Amy was lucky, because her parents were diligent. But other parents of PKU children start to become lax about the diet after developmental milestones are passed — when the youngsters start walking and talking like the other children on the block. By this time, children are also more adventuresome, getting cookies from the cookie jar or an apple from a well-meaning neighbor. Both items, however, are rich in phenylalanine. If the parents are lax or the child sneaks food, no one can tell. Noncompliance with the diet does not result in visible effects, as would noncompliance with insulin when a person goes into a diabetic shock. With PKU such problems as learning difficulties or hyperactivity show up only years later.

Who is responsible for seeing that a child remains on the diet during these early formative years? The parents? The physician? The state? Dr. Allen Crocker, who follows 170 PKU families in his Boston clinic, said that he has never gone to court over noncompliance, but that such action would not be without precedent. "If a family mismanaged juvenile diabetes, we wouldn't hesitate to take legal action to separate the child from the family. Letting a child go into shock just because the family couldn't get their act together would be criminal."

But how far can a family be coerced into following the diet, especially since medical researchers are still pondering how long to keep children on it? No definitive answers have been reached; just a series of suppositions. It is thought that only growing brain cells are affected by high phenylalanine rates. Is it therefore safe to stop the diet when the child is four, when brain cells have stopped growing?

In a recent study at the Johns Hopkins Hospital in Baltimore, four-year-olds with PKU were studied over a two-year period. One group of youngsters was weaned from the special diet; the other continued on the restricted menu. The children who remained on the diet gained more weight than did those eating whatever they wished, but height gains were the same for the two groups, and the more important test scores, those for intellectual and motor abilities, were similar.

Although no harmful effects of stopping the diet were noted, findings are still preliminary. Should parents gamble that the early data are correct and stop treatment? Should they continue with a difficult regimen that may not be necessary? The answers probably will not be in for several years, yet parents have to start making decisions today. "I don't know what I would do about stopping the diet if I had a PKU child," said Elizabeth Walker, a nutritionist with the Maryland Health Department who counsels every PKU family in the state about the diet.

"With mass screening to identify as many PKU babies as possible, to treat them and have them grow up virtually normal, we are saving this generation, but what are we doing to the next one?" questioned Walker. Young girls with PKU grow up to be young women with PKU. The condition is no longer harmful to them — their brains are fully formed — but it will be harmful to any baby whom, for nine months, they flood with their naturally high phenylalanine levels. It is frightening to note that a large proportion of babies born to PKU mothers will be mentally retarded. PKU women also have many miscarriages — nature's way of preventing the full development of severely defective fetuses.

The alternative for maternal PKUs is sterilization, an assured but very restrictive way of not exposing a fetus to harmful levels of phenylalanine. Another alternative is to keep levels of the amino acid low by having the mother return to the special diet. But it is unknown at this time how much phenylalanine is needed for the fetus to grow normally and how much is toxic.

*

In-the-womb therapy raises many difficult and still-unanswerable questions, but it promises much. When April Murphy was born in November 1973, she had already been treated for three months for a rare metabolic disease that might have doomed her to an early death. Her sister had died at the age of three months, already severely retarded.

April and her sister suffered from a disorder known as methylmalonic acidemia (MMA), an abnormal buildup in the body of methylmalonic acid, which results in recurrent vomiting and mental and physical retardation — all because of defective synthesis of vitamin B_{12}. Without this synthesis there is not enough of the vitamin to serve as a co-enzyme in the breakdown of certain amino acids in the body. As a result, tremendous amounts of methylmalonic acid accumulate in the body fluids, and the damage begins.

If the genetic message to supply vitamin B_{12} is missing, why not provide it directly, by means of injections, suggested Dr. Mary G. Ampola of Tufts–New England Medical Center in Boston. Mrs. Murphy began receiving 5000 times the normal dose of vitamin B_{12} when she was thirty-two weeks pregnant — superdoses that would pass through the placenta barrier and saturate the tissues of the fetus.

When April was born, three months later, all signs indicated that the treatment had been successful. Although an analysis of April's first voided urine showed thirty times the amount of methylmalonic acid that is in the first voided urine of normal newborns, it was only $\frac{1}{1000}$ the average amount excreted by untreated babies with the vitamin deficiency.

After her birth, April was put on a very strict low-protein diet, one that eliminated the particular amino acids known to be harmful to her. She thrived on this diet and is still on it. In addition, she takes daily doses of the essential vitamin she lacks. She is plump, bright-eyed, cheerful, and, more important, she is developing normally.

Manipulating the uterine environment is a portent of things to come. Lives are saved, but each medical advance is based on a calculated risk of unknown proportions.

Sex Selection: A Misuse of Medical Advances

April's prenatal diagnosis and intrauterine treatments were risky, but the ethics of saving a life by attempting something new were compelling. It is less compelling to use prenatal-detection techniques for ethically questionable reasons.

Amniocentesis discloses the sex of a fetus, an important piece of information for carriers of sex-linked diseases like hemophilia. Each male infant has a 50 percent chance of having the disease; each female will be normal. Predicting sex is more than a crude therapeutic tool for weeding out hemophiliacs; it now unlocks information that has been sought for thousands of years. Hippocrates believed that males develop in the right uterine horn, females in the left. Accordingly, Aristotle counseled women desiring boy children to "think male," and to lie on their right side.

Over the millenniums, little has changed, and philosophers and physicians are still devising ways for a do-it-yourself system of sex preselection. Some systems rely on the timing of ejaculation, depth of penetration, or an acidic preintercourse douche if a girl is desired, an alkaline one for a boy.

Another controversial sex-selection system involves inseminating a woman artificially with sperm that have been specially processed in a patented solution that separates out the male-producing Y sperm, which are thought to be the strongest sperm swimmers. A concentration with a high percentage of male-producing sperm is then inserted into the female. According to the developers of this process, a male baby is produced nine times out of ten.

Using amniocentesis as a way of determining sex carries a steep price tag. To get this information, a woman must invest between $150 and $250 for the test and laboratory analysis. Further, she must pay for an abortion if she is carrying what she considers to be the "wrong" sex. The medical profession is uneasy about the implications of its newfound ability to detect sex for sex's sake. "There is no medical reason for it," one obstetrician-gynecologist said, "but if people have the right not to have children — based on the right to have an abortion — why can't they have the right not to have a boy or not to have a girl, as they wish?"

More and more genetic counselors and obstetricians are encountering requests for sex selection. Some couples use fake histories; others seek out physicians who believe abortion for sex determination is acceptable.

One pregnant woman and her husband came to a genetic-counseling clinic reporting a family history of hemophilia and seeking prenatal diagnostic services. After the amniocentesis, their physician gave them good news: there was no danger of hemophilia, because the woman was going to have a girl. The couple, however, were not as delighted as the physician. They had two girls at home and wanted a boy. The story about being at risk for hemophilia was concocted as a ruse to get information about the fetus's sex. They chose to have an abortion.

Amniocentesis for sex selection is viewed by some physicians as a way of saving a life. Take the hypothetical case of thirty-year-old Sally Trimble. She and her husband have two boys and do not want to have a large family. She becomes pregnant by accident and plans to have an abortion. But then she has second thoughts: "Wouldn't it be nice to have a girl. I would continue with this pregnancy if I knew for sure I was going to have a girl."

In this circumstance, if Sally has amniocentesis for sex determination, it would save a life because she would have an abortion — 100 percent chance of no baby — unless she learns the sex of the fetus. If she does have the test, however, she reduces by 50 percent her chance of having an abortion.

There are no reliable data on how often amniocentesis is used for sex selection, but the general feeling among obstetricians-gynecologists is that it does take place. When a number of genetic counselors were polled by a leading geneticist and baldly asked whether they would recommend prenatal detection to allow parents to choose the sex, with the understanding that a fetus of "unwanted sex" would be intentionally aborted, 15 percent responded yes.

Most genetic counselors are adamant about not doing amniocentesis for women like Sally Trimble. "Abortion for sex selection tends to trivialize medical technological advances. Sex is not a disease that can be treated," John Fletcher argued.

"We give all our priorities for amniocentesis for people at risk with diseases," said Howard University geneticist Dr. Robert Murray, pointing out that each year there are more than 200,000 women who need prenatal studies, yet barely 4000 get to have an amniocentesis. "It is still a scarce resource," Murray continued, "and it should not be flagrantly wasted."

Ethical problems with sex determination will become more acute as new methods — cheaper, more accessible, less risky — are developed. It is predicted that a simple blood test early in pregnancy will be able to indicate fetal sex. Reports from China indicate that an analysis of cells shed into the cervical canal in early stages of pregnancy can provide an accurate indication of sex. This test is being done, according to a Chinese medical journal, "to help women who desire family planning." And here is how some families were planned in the Manchurian city of Anshan: of fifty-three women carrying males, only one chose to terminate the pregnancy. Two thirds of the forty-six women carrying females elected to have abortions.

Preference for male children is virtually a global desire. It is estimated that there would be a 20 percent excess of male births if all parents had their way. The implications of this — ethical, economic, cultural, sociological — are enormous. Since men commit most of the crimes, would our already hazardous streets become more dangerous? In a more positive vein, we know that by the time we reach sixty-five, there are normally seven males to every ten females. Would more men eliminate some of the prospects of lonely widowhood for older women?

While it is possible that sex choices will be made, it is not likely to be a universal movement. Rather, it will, in the words of a Princeton medical sociologist, be "limited to a small hard core of couples who have had four or five girls and are knocking themselves out to get a boy."

The genetic make-up of each individual is just beginning to be uncoded, and, at least initially, knowledge about predispositions has helped more than it has harmed. Fatal diseases are being avoided, and youngsters doomed to mental and physical retardation are living healthy and happy lives. The same genetic-detection tools, however, can be used to stigmatize healthy carriers of a disease, or to select an heir for a male-less family. Technology delivers only the ability to decipher genetic messages: how wisely and well this information is used is left to each one of us.

Chapter 4

Tomorrow's Genetics

DAVID CAMP is alive today because a billion bone marrow cells, taken from the hip of his sister Doreen, were injected into his own body when he was an infant. David was born with an immune-deficiency disease, and, like all the twelve male children on his mother's side of the family, he was marked for an early death. The course of his genetic heritage was changed radically as his sister's cells were incorporated into his body to provide the immunologic system he originally lacked.

When Larry Newell was three years old, he had trouble seeing and couldn't distinguish one color from another. Doctors found a cancerous tumor and removed his left eye. Larry's son John developed the same eye cancer, retinoblastoma, when he was fifteen months old, and he too had his eye removed. It is likely that John's children will fall victim to this inherited form of cancer. Aggressive treatment such as removing an eye keeps people like the Newells alive.

And April Murphy survived infancy because her rare vitamin deficiency was treated so early in life. Even before she was born April received supplements for the vitamin she needed to prevent a lethal buildup of methylmalonic acid.

Addition, subtraction, deletion, replacement. Special diets, drugs, surgery, transplants. These are the ways that children are treated for genetic defects today. But changes are underway, and researchers are working on ways to get at the root cause of genetic diseases by supplying not the missing substance but the enzyme that is responsible for making that substance.

Dr. Roscoe Brady, of the National Institutes of Health, is isolating enzymes from human placentas and injecting them in patients who are missing them. Brady's innovative and award-winning work involves the lipid-degrading enzymes that are deficient in patients with Gaucher's and Fabry's diseases.

New lipid materials are formed continuously in the human body, and the older lipids must be degraded or eliminated to make room. In Gaucher's patients, however, lipid accumulation is usually four times above normal levels. Within seventy-two hours after an enzyme injection, Brady reports, lipid levels drop to normal, and the unrelenting pain, in the bones and joints, where the lipids concentrate, diminishes. Supplying the enzyme does not alter the course of the disease — yet. It is only a temporary measure, and, although lipid levels rise again, they never reach their preinjection highs.

Brady is concerned with the unknown factors involved in his research. If one dose removes 25 percent of the accumulated lipids, would four times that dose remove 100 percent? Would it be safe or toxic? Should he try it? Is it ethical not to try? "I have five hundred letters from people who are in pain, people who are trying to overcome the constant use of habit-forming painkilling drugs like morphine," Brady said.

Enzyme shots won't stop the disease once it is in progress. The pain is halted temporarily; then it begins again. But if the enzyme injections were given before the damage began, could they prevent the damage from ever occurring?

"Metabolism in the brain has its greatest period of activity during the first few months of life," Brady explained. "If we could get the enzyme into a person with an enzyme deficiency during those critical early months of life, then we might be able to eliminate some of the effects of genetic diseases."

But he can only hypothesize that injecting the missing Tay-Sachs enzyme early in infancy — even prenatally — could prevent the tragic birth of a child like Joann. Since the blood-brain barrier prevents materials from passing from one to the other, the enzyme missing in Tay-Sachs babies would not be able to reach the rapidly growing brain cells even if such an injection of enzymes were available.

Medical researchers are trying to find ways to open the blood-brain barrier without causing paralysis. There is some indication that the barrier may be open in infancy, which means that there *may* be time for an injection of the missing Tay-Sachs enzyme to act effectively before destruction of the central nervous system begins.

A break through the blood-brain barrier, coupled with advances in synthesizing enzymes and injecting them, holds great promise for treating genetic diseases. But even with effective enzyme replacements, problems of genetic diseases are not erased. Enzymes cannot replicate themselves, and periodic reinjections will be needed. The disease may be in control for the lifetime of the victim, but it will not be eradicated. It is still there — imprinted indelibly on each gene.

Changing the Aberrant Gene

For long-lasting alterations in the treatment and occurrence of genetic diseases, changes must be made at the genetic level. But the notion of altering genes raises hopes as well as fears. "A lot of people are afraid of molecules that can carry out exponential growth and get out of control. But that is life, after all. Perhaps people are just afraid of life," said Dr. Carl Merrill, a molecular biologist at the NIH who has reproduced enzymes in genes.

"Our society is based on genetic engineering," he went on. "Selective breeding has been used for millenniums; domesticated animals, crops, even the green revolution, make use of basic genetic-engineering principles."

Genetic engineering is concerned not with the inception of life but with the method of transmitting life. It includes conception by artificial insemination, treatment of diseases *in utero*, and the ultimate — the manufacture of a human being to exact specifications. Genetic engineering also has the potential to cure many of the genetic diseases discussed in this book. Through the alteration of genes, the error for sickle cell anemia in hemoglobin or the genetic mistake that inhibits phenylalanine metabolism could be corrected. Consider the following genetic scheme for sickle cell disease linked to a basic concept of genetics: turning genetic action on and off.

Humans make different hemoglobins at different times of their lives. The hemoglobin made during fetal days (HbF) switches, by some unknown genetic mechanism, to adult hemoglobin (HbA). At birth, an infant's hemoglobin is still 60 to 80 percent HbF, but by four months the switch to adult hemoglobin has taken place. Researchers now know that sickling takes place only in adult hemoglobin cells. In the early months of life, babies who will probably become sickle cell victims are protected from sickling damage by the presence of the fetal hemoglobin.

If the shift from HbF to HbA were prevented — by inserting a regulatory gene to dampen the production of adult hemoglobin — then sickle cell disease could be conquered. Researchers already know that adults can live with fetal hemoglobin. Some people, curiously, keep on producing fetal hemoglobin, and there are a few known cases of adults who never make the switch to HbA. They nonetheless are normal, healthy, and have neither anemia nor any other blood abnormalities.

The clue to the hemoglobin switch is not known yet. Should researchers continue exploring the mysteries of the genetic code to get the answer, or is it too risky?

*

A worldwide ethical debate was triggered when three little sisters in West Germany were inoculated with a live virus that was thought to carry the gene for the synthesis of an enzyme, arginase, that the girls were missing. Without this enzyme, an amino acid called arginine builds up in the blood stream, resulting in severe mental retardation, spastic paraplegia, and epileptic seizures. The girls were hopelessly ill, and the damage done by the amino acid buildup was probably irreversible.

The virus they were given, Shope papilloma virus (SPV), was discovered by Dr. Richard E. Shope of the Rockefeller Institute in 1930. This virus, Shope reported, produced some strange characteristics. When injected with the virus, cottontail rabbits developed huge horny warts on their skin, and when Dr. Shope injected himself with it, his serum arginine levels fell, and remained depressed for years. He died thirty-three years later at the age of sixty-four, of cancer, and his mentor, the Nobel laureate F. Peyton Rous, who was also exposed to the virus, died at ninety — also of cancer.

In the early 1970s, Dr. Heinz Georg Terheggen, a pediatrician in Cologne, knowing the danger of malignancy from the virus and the irreversible nature of genetic therapy, injected the three girls with a shot of SPV. Researchers around the world began to debate the ethics of using a dangerous and poorly understood genetic maneuver in a clinical setting.

Medical World News canvassed its readers on the ethical issues of gene therapy for the German girls, and nearly 80 percent of the physicians responding were in favor of going ahead with the therapy if the parents consented. The physicians reasoned that if nothing happened or if the patients grew worse, then the treatments will have failed. But what if the girls' arginine levels returned to normal? Even if the damage done was irreversible, normal arginine levels could arrest progression of the disease. And other children born with the deficiency could benefit from this experiment and have the opportunity for a normal life — if they received injections of the virus right after birth, perhaps even while in the womb.

The three girls were inoculated, but their concentrations of arginine failed to drop. Dr. Terheggen believes that the virus failed to synthesize arginase in the youngsters, though it had done so in Dr. Shope and dozens of other laboratory workers, because the virus he used for the girls had deteriorated during storage.

Some medical researchers think that Terheggen was lucky that the virus had degraded; it might have done considerable harm if it had been active. Terheggen, however, turns aside the ethical objections. He said, "What we are doing — using a virus as a vector for genetic information — is gene therapy, not gene manipulation."

Gene therapy still does not mean cure. Even if the three German girls had responded positively to the gene action in the SPV, they would still have the mutant gene that prevented the enzyme synthesis in the first place, a mutant gene they could pass on to their offspring. Gene therapy, if all goes well, is for the patients' lifetime, not for the lifetime of their progeny.

*

Basic questions about gene therapy — its safety, its efficacy, and its limits — are still unanswered. Yet research on it proceeds. Carl Merrill, for example, is working on a genetic route to produce the missing enzyme for a disease in which patients become mentally retarded because they cannot process the milk sugar, galactose, properly. Merrill has grown cells from a patient with galactosemia, as the enzyme deficiency is called, in tissue culture in his NIH laboratory. When he infected the culture with a bacterial virus carrying the gene for the missing enzyme, human cells from the galactosemic patient began producing it. This work, which has so far taken place in the lab, may eventually move along the traditional developmental route — from laboratory, to animal and human experimentation, to clinical use.

At the Massachusetts Institute of Technology, Dr. Har Gobind Khorana, who won the Nobel Prize for deciphering the genetic code, created the first workable artificial gene, in 1977, by linking together tiny bits of chemicals into an exact copy of a bacterial gene. He then transplanted it to a living bacterium and watched it function as a "real" gene. Khorana can do something with his artificial gene that he cannot do with a real one: he can manipulate the gene's functioning, its stop, go, and other control mechanisms.

The goal of the experiment is not to correct genetic defects, but rather to learn more about the gene itself and how it is regulated. But once this is known, genetic diseases may be amenable to treatment by the substitution of healthy, artificial genes for defective ones.

Khorana's work, at least so far, involves making a gene that is already present in all living cells. It is confined to one gene only, to one species only. But the techniques could be used to introduce into an organism a gene that does not naturally occur there, thus raising the same potential for hazard as recombinant DNA.

The controversial recombinant DNA work joins — or recombines — naturally occurring genes from different species. The genes from one organism are transplanted to another, giving the latter new, and possibly unpredictable, abilities.

With such recombination and transplantation of DNA (deoxyribonucleic acid) — the tiny chemical strands on which genetic code is imprinted — it may be possible to change the genes of plants, animals, and human beings, manipulating them at will. Human insulin for diabetics, clotting factor for hemophiliacs, and the missing enzymes that cause so many of the genetic diseases could be produced by attaching genes for these properties to bacterial viruses and letting them grow. Critics of recombinant DNA, however, talk about the risks of viruses escaping from the laboratory and multiplying in human hosts.

Separate buildings, air locks, protective clothing, and showering are features of the strictest levels of physical containment of recombinant DNA material. But there are no guarantees that these precautions will always be successful. Of the 5000 laboratory-acquired infections recorded over the last thirty years, one-third occurred in labs with special containment facilities, according to *Science*. At the army's former biological warfare laboratories in Fort Detrick in Frederick, Maryland — the place the National Institutes of Health selected to perform its recombinant DNA experiments — even though there were strict levels of containment, there were more than 400 cases of infection and three deaths over twenty-five years. The precautions taken for facilities devoted solely to research on recombinant DNA, however, are even more stringent.

The risks versus the benefits: Will the cure be worse than the disease? No one has the answers, but the debate on genetic manipulation precipitated a flood of questions about the role of scientific and medical research. Should it be done? What precautions should be taken? Who should do the monitoring? What are the limits to its use?

This far-reaching debate started in the laboratories of prestigious medical research institutions and medical schools; it attracted public interest through town meetings, television, and newspaper coverage; it spread to city councils and state legislatures in areas where recombinant DNA research laboratories were being built, and on to the U.S. Congress, where ways were sought to control DNA research.

The DNA debate opened the public's eyes to the benefits as well as dangers of the increasing ability to change our genetic make-up, far more than did mass screenings in the ghetto for sickle cell anemia or in Jewish community centers for Tay-Sachs disease. Recombinant DNA cuts across ethnic and racial lines, and it potentially affects every living being.

Mapping Genes and Recharting the Future

Genetics is like the proverbial iceberg: only the tip of the enormous mass is immediately apparent. Techniques developed today for relatively rare diseases or for esoteric research have potential applicability to major life-threatening diseases.

"The big issue in genetics is not cloning or enzyme replace-

ment or even recombinant DNA," explains Dr. Neil Holtzman of Johns Hopkins, "but rather ways to translate screening, detection, and the treatment of rare diseases to the major
killers. For example, one person in twenty-five is a carrier
for cystic fibrosis, and it is likely that one day we will be able
to identify CF carriers. Genetic counseling for diseases in the
future will mean counseling about the big diseases."

*

"Currently we can identify only a small group of individuals
with certain rare diseases," said Dr. Fred H. Bergmann, director of the genetics program at the National Institute of
General Medical Sciences. "But add them up and they become a significant number of people. There are probably
more papers written about Lesch-Nyhan syndrome than there
are people with the disease, but it has taught us a lot about
genetic deficiencies and how to identify them, all of which
could be helpful in working out genetic markers."

Geneticists are beginning to identify the location of human
genes and, though most of the map of human genetics is still
uncharted, more than 200 human genes have been assigned
locations on a chromosome. The goal is to identify all of the
thousands of human genes that determine hereditary traits.
When the map is complete, it will theoretically be possible
for researchers to screen for every physical disease with a
genetic link — from relatively rare conditions, such as Huntington's disease, to the major killers, heart disease and cancer.

*

The number one cause of death, heart disease, does not hit
as arbitrarily as it seems. Heart disease has genetic roots, and
if people who are predisposed to coronary problems because
of their genes are identified and treated in early childhood,
decades could be added to their lives. Atherosclerosis — the
buildup of fatty deposits, which narrows arteries and can lead
eventually to heart attacks in middle-aged adults — begins
in childhood. In a study of 100 families in which one parent

suffered a heart attack, researchers found that nearly a third of the 250 children in these families had significantly high blood fats. It is expected that at least 50 percent of these youngsters will have heart attacks when they get older.

One out of 500 Americans has a genetic condition in which the cells are deficient in cholesterol receptors. These receptors normally suppress cholesterol synthesis. For a person with this condition, hypercholesterolemia, the fatty deposits build up in the blood, clog arteries, and often cause heart attack by the time he or she is forty. If both parents have the defective gene and pass it on, coronary heart disease is likely to develop in their children in adolescence or even earlier. These youngsters have a grim future: survival past the age of thirty has not been reported among people who inherit the gene from both parents.

*

One out of four people now living will develop cancer at some point in his or her life. Can it be predicted? Is cancer written on each individual's genetic code? Research on the genetics of cancer is just beginning, but already more than 160 genetic conditions have been identified as causing either a malignant or premalignant tumor.

There are three genetic causes for cancer.

❰Inheriting the gene for it: Larry Newell's eye cancer, retinoblastoma, is an example of a single gene defect, and each of his children has a 50 percent chance of getting the disease.

❰Having many genes interact with environmental factors: A nonsmoker's chance of dying of lung cancer is four times greater than the average if a close relative also has lung cancer. Combining that genetic predisposition with an environmental factor — smoking — radically increases the risks; a smoker related to a lung cancer victim has a chance of dying of lung cancer fourteen times greater than the nonsmoker.

❰Having a chromosomal abnormality: The incidence of leukemia in Down's syndrome children is eleven times greater than in nonmongoloids. And the incidence of breast cancer in men with an extra female chromosome (XXY) is sixty-six times greater than in normal males. When pieces of genetic material on the chromosomes are either absent or present in excess, there is also an increased chance of a person's getting cancer. Most patients with chronic myelocytic leukemia, for example, have a distinct chromosomal peculiarity: part of one chromosome is translocated to another, and it is thought that when the exchange takes place, some genetic material is lost. It is not the translocation but the deletion that is thought to cause cancer.

"When we have a fully completed genetic map, we will be able to determine at birth what a person will die of," Bergmann said. "But that is just data. Individuals will need a better understanding of what the statistics mean to their lives. Does it mean you will automatically drop dead of a heart attack at forty-five if you are genetically predisposed to early myocardial infarction, or does it offer you an option of altering your lifestyle?"

Many people still think that if a disease or condition is genetic, then it is predetermined that they will get sick and possibly die from it, and that there is nothing they can do about it. Bergmann disagrees with this philosophy. "This assumes a Calvinistic predetermination that is ridiculous. There is no point in screening and knowing about your disease potential unless you are going to do something about it. We already alter our environment to avoid certain diseases — taking vitamin C to avoid scurvy, putting PKU children on low-phenylalanine diets. We now have to learn how to alter our environment to avoid the more pervasive diseases."

*

There is a fine line between being at risk and accepting the finality of that risk. Following the proper diet, giving up smoking, and exercising wisely can change a genetic tendency to heart attacks. If a woman is marked to have diabetes and knows about it, she can take steps to prevent her getting the disease. Avoiding sugar, eating few starches, and watching calories would be essential, because even a 15 percent increase over a recommended weight could trigger the disease. Is it worth the trauma of a lifelong restricted diet to fight against a genetic marker?

Being too vigilant about genetic predisposition can, ironically, cause problems. If a man has a family history of lung cancer, will there be more risks than benefits reaped from his getting repeated x-rays to catch and treat the disease early? Will his vigilance — getting x-rays — provoke the genetically determined precancerous cells into becoming malignant ones?

Consider the dilemma of Karen McGinty, nineteen years old and destined by her genetic make-up to have breast cancer. Her two sisters developed it when they were twenty-two and twenty-nine, respectively. Her mother was diagnosed as having breast cancer at the age of forty-two, her maternal grandmother at forty-eight, and several maternal aunts and cousins developed it during their forties and fifties.

Karen's physician recommended that she have a double mastectomy, with synthetic breasts inserted in flaps under her skin. An extreme measure, perhaps, but, given her genetic predisposition, the only other choices were very risky: monthly self-examination in which only already well-formed cancers are usually detected, and having her breasts x-rayed twice a year to check for cancer — a procedure that might result in a significant accumulation of radiation exposure throughout her lifetime. Her susceptibility to breast cancer might also interact with the radiation exposure and possibly cause a heightened risk of a malignant tumor. What should Karen do?

Theresa Boyd was substantially older when she finally made her decision to have a double mastectomy. She was forty-five and previously had had several cysts and benign tumors removed from her breasts. Her family history of breast cancer was grim. Her sister, mother, and aunt all died from it before they were fifty. Theresa felt doomed, until she had both of her breasts removed even though malignant tumors were never detected. "I talked it over with my husband, and we both came to the conclusion that it was far more important that I don't develop it [breast cancer] than that I have breasts.

"I feel relieved for the first time since my sister died," said Theresa after her operation. "I saw the family pattern and knew that I was next in line to get breast cancer and have an early death. It was a difficult decision — breasts are so idolized in our society — but I took control over my destiny."

As widespread as cancer is, there are few people experienced in genetic counseling for it. It seems strange that counselors are more attuned to statistical risks for Tay-Sachs, PKU, and even rarer diseases, such as Lesch-Nyhan.

Data are beginning to be collected about cancer-prone families. There is more than a threefold increased risk for a person's getting a site-specific cancer — breast, stomach, colon, prostate gland, lung — if a close relative has had that kind of cancer. Although taking a genetic history is far from routine practice with most physicians, knowing about a genetic predisposition and failing to act on it — whether it be for a rare enzyme deficiency or for cancer — could be considered malpractice.

*

Screening for the big genetic diseases raises many of the same questions as does screening for the rare ones. Should everyone know his or her genetic make-up? Should all conditions be screened, or only those for which treatment is available?

Mass screening for heart disease, for example, is not recommended since correct treatment is disputed. There is no proof that following a low-cholesterol diet will ensure that the dieter will not have premature heart disease. Heart attacks have occurred in people who have perfectly normal, even low, serum cholesterol levels. In fact, no threshold has been established below which heart disease is not known to occur.

Complicating the issue, only one of the genetic forms of heart disease — hypercholesterolemia — is easily detectable in the period right after birth, and even then, high cholesterol levels do not necessarily mean early death. Most of the infants with high blood cholesterol levels found in their umbilical cords have normal levels when they are retested a year later.

The problem lies not only in screening, but also in what to do with the information gleaned from it. If there is an indication of high cholesterol, when should treatment start? Lesions caused by deposits of cholesterol may or may not be more readily reversed with early treatment, but it is clearly too late to halt the process in a forty-year-old.

In severe cases, drug therapy is needed, but once it is started it must remain a lifelong process. Should the expensive medication, which is known to cause gallstones, be taken daily for many years to prevent possible development of severe atherosclerosis or a heart attack that might occur decades later?

Victims of hypercholesterolemia can also try a new concept in prolonging life: a dialysislike machine that removes the cholesterol from the blood of patients with high levels of the fatty substance. This machine, which would do its cholesterol removing two to three times weekly, could be as important to victims of coronary artery disease as dialysis is to kidney patients. But this is yet another example of high-cost halfway technology designed to counter a genetic condition, not to cure it.

*

There is a bothersome Big Brother aspect of knowing all there is to know about each person's genetic make-up. "There will be a big data file of all your genetic troubles," warned

Dr. Bergmann, "and this has all the potential for misuse." Bergmann is concerned because he foresees genetic profiles for each person — a basic profile being issued for each baby at birth, with updating and expanding as the child grows and more precise tests come out of research labs.

"There have to be safeguards against this tricky time bomb," he cautioned. "Whenever there are innovations, there are troubles. For every fix there is a new problem."

Some people are already getting the Big Brother once-over, with threats of pre-employment genetic screening, losing out on high-paying jobs if they "fail." This is similar to what happened to blacks who were identified as having sickle cell trait.

There is a form of pulmonary emphysema associated with an inherited deficiency of a serum enzyme called alpha-1-antitrypsin. Nearly 50 percent of the patients under fifty years of age who are hospitalized with emphysema have this deficiency, according to a study in a Veterans' Administration hospital. Although this does not mean that all men and women with the deficiency will have respiratory problems, a pre-employment test in factories where industrial chemicals are used — chemicals to which people with respiratory problems are particularly sensitive — could identify people with this deficiency and restrict their job freedom accordingly. Employers could assign them to jobs in areas where risks are lowest — and for which the pay is likely to be the lowest.

Consider another genetically linked condition and its effect on careers. There is a strong relationship between a chronic but treatable arthritis of the lower spine, ankylosing spondylitis, and the presence of a B_{27} antigen, a specific antibody-producing agent. Ninety percent of the people with the disease have the antigen, but no more than 20 percent of those in the general population with the antigen will develop the disorder.

Should people with B_{27} antigen avoid professions that are likely to place an excessive strain on their back — being a surgeon or a professional football player — just because they might develop a disease that is, after all, treatable? Could knowing too much about genetic predispositions be a curse instead of a help?

*

Genetic messages are indelibly imprinted, but human beings are so malleable that they can change their coded destiny with a variety of tricks — from sophisticated technology to common-sense diets and exercise programs. Medical technological advances give information that can be used or abused. There can be gains or losses with the new ability to create life and manipulate it.

Genetic research is in its infancy. More clues to our destinies and how they can be altered genetically will be uncovered. But there is much that can be learned from the past successes and failures as the discoveries of prenatal detection and early treatment of rare diseases from the past twenty-five years are applied to more common diseases in the next twenty-five years. Problems once faced by thousands will have to be resolved by millions.

II

LIFE

Chapter 5

Muddled Medical Decisions

MEDICAL DECISIONS are made on inconclusive evidence — every day, with every patient. The attractive technological advances of the past two decades still provide only limited information, and predictive powers remain unreliable. Yet in spite of these limitations and uncertainties, decisions must be made continually about the sick and the healthy, the young and the old, the newly born and the dying.

Compounding the problem, medical decisions are increasingly influenced by nonmedical considerations. An eighty-year-old terminally ill woman, ridden with cancer, is not allowed to take narcotic pain medications because the doctor fears she will become addicted. Is her treatment — or lack of it — based on sound medical principles, or on the physician's moral values?

When thirty-two-year-old Allan Barnes was admitted to the hospital with a recurrent skin tumor, which had affected the lymph nodes draining the area, he was faced with the dilemma of not knowing which course of treatment to follow. The surgeon suggested surgery, and the immunologist recommended immunological treatment. Surgery didn't seem like much of a cure to Barnes. Though the new tumor could be removed, another would probably appear in a short time. Immunological treatment — injecting experimental drugs directly into the malignant tissue — would inhibit the growth of tumor cells, if all went well. But if the experiment failed, Barnes would likely die. Now he, the patient, had to make a decision that involved a choice between medical values and moral values — between surgery and the certainty of a short life span, or immunology and the possibility of a longer life. Which treatment should he choose?

Choosing a treatment for breast cancer provides another example of the uncertainties inherent in medical decision-making. For decades, a radical mastectomy — removal of the entire breast and chest muscles plus underarm lymph nodes — was the standard way for treating breast cancers. Questions about the efficacy of radical mastectomies were rarely asked.

Today, cancer experts and women's health groups are questioning the high rate at which radical mastectomies are done. Dr. William Stewart Halsted, an innovator, in 1890, of the radical mastectomy technique, "would be the last person today to accept the continued use of [it] without question," Dr. Vincent T. DeVita, director of the Division of Cancer Treatment at the National Cancer Institute, reported to Senator Edward M. Kennedy during congressional hearings on the progress in treatment of breast cancer.

Halsted envisioned the procedure as a way of controlling large and very advanced tumors of the breast, in which the cancer often had spread to underarm lymph nodes. But now, with early diagnosis of breast cancer by super x-rays called mammographies, tiny tumors that can be neither felt nor seen with the naked eye are being discovered. Some of these tumors are so small that it is difficult for pathologists to do accurate biopsies on them. (The ethical problems associated with diagnostic advances are discussed in further detail in Chapter 7.) Halsted rarely detected small tumors, since early diagnosis was virtually unheard of. "Surely, Halsted would have questioned whether a radical procedure was necessary for such patients," concluded DeVita.

In spite of this sobering insight, the radical mastectomy is the treatment performed on most of the American women with breast cancer — a medical choice based on a tradition established without a clear-cut justification. Yet there are several ways of treating breast cancer — local removal of the tumor, modified mastectomy in which the breast is removed but the underarm muscles remain, radiation treatments, and chemotherapy — each of which may be as effective as radical mastectomy in patients with early-detected breast cancer. Treatment is moving from a standardized approach that calls for every patient to have a radical, to custom-tailored therapies designed to fit the precise characteristics of the cancer and the patient who harbors it.

Is choosing a lumpectomy — the removal of just the tumor and not the entire breast — a medical decision or a quality-of-life decision? Given all the conflicting information about breast cancer treatments, how can any decision — medical, moral, or a combination of the two — be made about which therapy to choose? Women cannot wait for the definitive answers. Decisions have to be made today — based on the available but inconclusive evidence.

Making moral decisions about medical issues is a burden that more and more patients and their families are bearing. They are no longer willing to give up their moral rights when they seek and receive medical care.

Questioning Medical Opinions

Gaby Lewis was four years old when her pediatrician suspected that she had epilepsy. He prescribed a rare drug for her "condition," and her father dutifully went to the pharmacy to have the prescription filled.

Mr. Lewis had gone to two drug stores, neither of which had that particular drug, before he began to question why he was prepared to give his daughter a medication that was so rare that popular pharmacies didn't carry it. Was Gaby's pediatrician — a specialist in well-baby care — qualified to make the diagnosis of epilepsy and to prescribe a drug for it?

It turned out that he wasn't. A pediatric neurologist whom Gaby's parents subsequently consulted confirmed neither the diagnosis of epilepsy nor the need for the potent and dangerous drug.

Gaby was lucky. Her parents were persistent, and she never took the drug. Most Americans, however, fail to question what is prescribed, and willingly take forty billion tablets, capsules, and other forms of medicine each year. As a result, some 300,000 men, women, and children suffer such severe adverse drug reactions annually that they have to be hospitalized, and some 18,000 die from the drugs' side effects. Moreover — and sadly — many patients become ill from the drugs without getting any benefits from them, because the drugs are either wrongly prescribed or incorrectly taken. The effect of an antibiotic, for example, is considerably weakened when it is taken on a full stomach. It is estimated that 10,000 Americans suffer life-threatening reactions each year solely from antibiotics that were unnecessarily prescribed.

"The average doctor tends to overprescribe: he orders unnecessary medicines, the wrong medicines, and too many medicines for the same illness," is part of the indictment by the HEW Task Force on Drug Prescribers.

"The system is a very sloppy one," agreed Stanley Jones, director of program planning at the Institute of Medicine and former staff director of Senator Edward M. Kennedy's Subcommittee on Health and Scientific Research. "Drugs are called safe and efficacious when they are released on the market. But this means that they are safe and efficacious for certain conditions only. Barbiturates, for example, are approved by the FDA for use by epileptics, but more than ninety-nine percent of the prescriptions for barbiturates are not for epileptics.

"We delegate responsibility for medical care to our physicians, who in turn base their decision on the FDA's saying a certain drug is safe. We think that the physicians are prescribing something safe, even if it is not so in the situation in which it will be used," Jones emphasized.

*

The doctor's word about drugs is not the only thing being questioned by concerned people. Patients who are advised to undergo surgery are also beginning to raise questions. A special report of the House Interstate and Foreign Commerce Committee, "The Cost and Quality of Health Care: Unnecessary Surgery," estimated that out of the fourteen million elective operations performed each year, 17 percent or 2.4 million, are unnecessary. These unnecessary procedures cost a staggering $4 billion. Not only is this costly financially; it is also costly in lives: there are 12,000 deaths a year attributed to these unnecessary operations.

The operation most frequently performed in the U.S. — the hysterectomy — rose a staggering 25 percent between 1970 and 1975, without a reported increase in diseased wombs. One million operations to remove the uterus are performed annually, many as a means of contraception or as a way to prevent any chance of future womb cancer. Testifying before a congressional committee on the excesses of surgery, Dr. James Sammons, executive vice president of the American Medical Association, defended the use of hysterectomies for women who had either a phobia about cancer or "acute pregnophobia." Are millions of women really so terrified of having uterine cancer or becoming pregnant that they willingly undergo a major operation that is not only risky but that also affects a basic aspect of their sexuality? Or are they relinquishing the right to make medical decisions about their own bodies?

Or consider tonsillectomies, performed since 600 B.C. with little proof of efficacy. The majority of the 900,000 tonsillectomies done each year in the U.S. are unnecessary or downright harmful; several hundred are lethal. "The factors behind a decision to operate appear to range from medical school preconceptions to attitudes derived from personal clinical experience or from financial concerns," said University of Pittsburgh pediatrician Jack L. Paradise. An indication of the different attitudes toward the operation is given by the statistics for two adjoining Massachusetts communities. In one, 65 percent of the children eventually have their tonsils removed; in the other, only 18 percent of the children have the operation.

The symptoms that cause doctors to recommend an appendectomy — a "popular" operation that more than 300,000 Americans have each year — are so vague, and surgeons so quick to operate, that up to 20 percent of the appendixes removed are normal, a figure that is considered acceptable. In fact, delaying an operation in the face of minor symptoms has been condemned in standard surgical textbooks.

A group of pediatricians at the Johns Hopkins University Medical School became concerned about appendectomies that were done as a matter of course on youngsters when the diagnosis of appendicitis was only vague and tentative. More than 92 percent of the children admitted to their hospital ward with suspected appendicitis were undergoing the operation. Then the pediatrics staff began examining the youngsters intensively — and periodically — waiting for a definitive diagnosis of appendicitis before operating. Under this vigilant plan, one quarter of the youngsters were sent home without having the operation. They had no further "stomach" problems or appendicitislike pains.

The ethics of whether, and when, to take out an appendix is indeed troublesome. "A patient has a pain in the right side. Do you take out the appendix immediately because it is convenient and you don't want to be bothered at two A.M. to do an operation? Or do you watch the patient carefully and monitor symptoms to avoid unnecessary surgery?" questioned New Haven surgeon Bernard Siegel. "Is scheduling the operation poor medicine, or is it prudent? If the operating room is heavily scheduled, you might not be able to get nurses or anesthesiologists at the time the appendix ruptures. While the patient will probably not die, because emergency measures are available, that patient could get much sicker than is necessary." Siegel does not have any answers to the questions he raised — but it is a hopeful sign that physicians are beginning to question the way they practice medicine.

Coronary care units (CCUs) also are under attack now, and their use is being scrutinized. Coronary care units are a reassuring concept to a person suffering a heart attack. In a CCU, every move, every heartbeat, is monitored twenty-four hours of each day. There are drugs, diagnostic tests, x-rays, electrocardiograms, and instant oxygen if breathing becomes difficult. With such vigilance, most patients think they will get better sooner than in the old days — before the advent of coronary care units and their fancy equipment.

It makes sense to think that CCUs will get frightened heart attack victims well faster, but it is not universally true, according to one hospital's records, published in the *Annals of Internal Medicine.* These data showed no difference, over a thirty-year period, in the mortality rate among heart attack victims, either in-hospital or after they had left the hospital. Think of it: thirty years of coronary care advances and no change in how the patient fares. Although one hospital's experiences cannot be generalized for the nation, it does challenge the unquestioned use of the CCU.

Maybe it would be better to stay at home? And that is just what a British report concluded: more patients survive heart attacks if they are treated at home than if they are hospitalized. A team of British physicians compared the records of nearly 2000 men who suffered heart attacks, half of whom were admitted to hospital coronary care units, the other half of whom were treated at home. At the end of nearly one year, the death rates were 20 percent among the patients treated at home, and 27 percent for those hospitalized.

Researchers theorize that it is a very anxiety-producing situation to be in a hospital, hooked up to sophisticated monitors that keep constant check on heart actions, and that this experience may cause more stress to the heart — and ultimately be responsible for extra deaths. The British group concludes that home care is better for many heart attack victims — but not for all. Those with persistent breathing problems, unrelieved pain, or other physiological symptoms need the attention and medical care available in hospitals.

The British report flies directly counter to the American approach. According to a Harvard Medical School specialist, "To send a patient home here [and not to the CCU] would almost be grounds for a malpractice suit." Since some patients might benefit from coronary care in hospitals and others might be harmed, what is needed is not a phasing out of CCUs but a more rational process of selecting which patients should go to them.

Since coronary care units are appropriate in many instances, they are unlikely to fall out of fashion. But the list of one-time accepted medical practices that have fallen out of fashion, if not into disgrace, is a long one, and it illustrates the fickleness of the practice of medicine. Consider just one example: gastric freezing.

During the 1960s, thousands of men and women underwent a procedure for treating ulcers before it was abandoned as useless. Patients swallowed an empty balloon with tubes attached to it. A coolant liquid, maintained at a constant below-freezing temperature by an $1800 hypothermia machine, entered the tubes and flowed into the balloon, which it continually irrigated for about an hour. The physiological principle involved in the procedure, popularly called gastric freezing, seemed to be a sound one, because lowering the stomach temperature temporarily reduces the secretion of acids that aggravates ulcers.

Gastric freezing was hailed in 1962 as a treatment for ulcer patients who would otherwise require surgery. It relieved pain, "significantly decreased" gastric secretions, and was safe, according to the surgeon who introduced the procedure. Contrast this to other methods for treating ulcers. Antacid drugs and special diets that had no long-lasting effects: they relieved symptoms only temporarily, and ulcers most often recurred. Another alternative, surgery, had a 10 percent mortality rate and a 10 percent recurrence rate among the lucky survivors. Given these options, it is not surprising that the initial reaction to gastric freezing was so positive.

Not everyone jumped on the bandwagon, and there were many physicians troubled by the lack of long-term evaluations and clinical trials of gastric freezing. Researchers began to question its efficacy and found that the percentage of patients reporting complete relief ranged widely, from 13 to 100 percent. Gastric freezing, researchers also found, did not affect long-term suppression of gastric secretions. There are other factors, such as stress, that must be considered in ulcer treatments. And then there was the possibility that patients receiving gastric freezing sought treatment when the disease was at its worst. The natural regression of the disease might have been mistakenly attributed to the effect of freezing.

By the end of the decade, gastric freezing was a has-been procedure. But the more than 2500 hypothermia machines that had been purchased — and used — were testimony to its temporary success.

Promising Help But Delivering Harm

Adding injury to insult, gastric freezing not only didn't help; it caused harm, including intestinal hemorrhaging. Numerous other popular procedures have caused great damage before falling out of favor. These are not isolated horror stories recorded in newspapers or professional journals. They are situations that stalk medical practice daily. "Iatrogenicity [adverse conditions caused by medical treatment], although it appears as a medical problem, is in reality a moral problem, and a particularly frustrating one," commented ethicist Albert Jonsen, of the University of California (San Francisco) School of Medicine. "Moral problems usually center on the question 'What should I do?' But this moral problem adds the perplexing phrase 'about the unforeseen and unintended consequences of my action.'"

Consider the plight of Gail Kalmowitz, introduced in

Chapter 1, blinded in early childhood because of life-saving treatment that she received at birth. Gail, born prematurely in 1953, was given treatment standard at the time: she was placed in an incubator with high concentrations of oxygen to help her breathe. In 1948, the American Academy of Pediatrics listed oxygen tanks as part of the standard equipment recommended for delivery rooms — in case a baby developed trouble breathing. "Oxygen should be administered to all premature infants immediately after birth," said the AAP in those days.

The eye condition that blinded Gail, retrolental fibroplasia (RLF), was first described in 1942, and its sudden appearance among low-birthweight babies was perplexing. No instances of the blinding condition were recorded in the years before oxygen-infused incubators were standard delivery-room equipment.

By 1949, RLF was estimated to be responsible for one third of the blind preschool children. By 1952, the year before Gail was born, it had reached epidemic proportions.

Medical researchers were looking for a cause of the condition. They eliminated the lights from the incubator and blood transfusions (which premature babies often require). Even cow's milk was questioned briefly. It was in this climate of uncertainty that the initial study of oxygen toxicity as a possible cause of RLF was published in 1952. "The pediatric community looked with great caution on this suggestion — as it did on any new concept that was not abundantly confirmed," according to *Pediatrics*, in a historical review of oxygen therapy and RLF. Physicians were also concerned because "restriction of much-needed oxygen might lead to tremendous harm, including brain damage or death."

But irrefutable data began to accumulate. Between 60 and 87 percent of the premature infants who received "routine" care with high oxygen concentrations for a month became blind; but only 20 to 35 percent of those who received low doses of oxygen for a short period of time developed the condition.

In 1955, when the AAP recommended limiting the use of oxygen in premature infants, the incidence of RLF immediately dropped, and the death rate of newborns rose. The costs of preventing retrolental fibroplasia were high: the AAP estimates that there were sixteen deaths for each sighted infant gained. The dilemma remains today, as medical technological advances permit smaller and smaller babies to survive after they are born prematurely. About half the babies born weighing two pounds or less will live, but half of these survivors will be blinded by RLF.

*

Another tragic iatrogenic condition is currently being discovered among teen-agers whose mothers took a drug to avert threatened miscarriages. The drug they were prescribed, diethylstilbestrol (DES), is now linked to cancer of the cervix or vagina in their daughters. There is also evidence that DES sons have genitourinary problems, such as a narrow urethral passage, which makes urinating difficult, abnormalities of the testes, and a low sperm count, and that the mothers themselves are at risk for breast cancer as well as other endocrine-related cancers — of the cervix, uterus, ovaries, and colon. Tragically, there was much harm but no benefit: the drug proved to be ineffective in preventing miscarriages.

From 1940 to the early 1970s, between 500,000 and two million pregnant women took DES or similar drugs. The odds that the daughters of these women will develop cancer because of their intrauterine exposures varies widely — from a low of one in 10,000 to a high of one in 1000. So far, more than fifty deaths have been attributed to a DES-associated vaginal or cervical cancer. Girls at risk undergo gynecological examinations starting at early ages, and they live with the constant dread of developing cancer. One overwrought eleven-year-old girl told her mother, after she had her first vaginal examination, "I'd rather die of cancer than go through that again." Her mother now worries more about the emotional scars left by DES and its aftermath than about the cancer.

While most DES daughters do not develop cancer, it is not uncommon for them to develop abnormal tissue growth called vaginal adenosis, which is like having the tissue that lines the inside of your mouth grow out onto your face. Although the tissue growth is healthy — initially, at least — it is misplaced. There is no solid proof that adenosis is a precursor of cancer, but many doctors are concerned because every time they see cancer of the vagina, they also see vaginal adenosis. It may be the bed from which cancers develop.

"I was devastated that a manmade factor that might have been avoided could cause cancer in my child," said Andrea Rago, a DES mother of a seven-year-old girl. "I thought they [the pills] would help me have the perfect baby, and I trusted that the doctor would only do what was good for me." Mrs. Rago, in fact, thought that the pills were vitamins. She had been especially careful about not taking drugs during her pregnancy. She stopped taking her regular course of allergy shots and refused to take even aspirin for minor ailments. But she dutifully took the red pills the physician prescribed for her, three times a day for three months.

Many DES mothers are still angry that they trusted their doctors, and are bitter that the drug they took was prescribed so freely before the verdict on its efficacy and safety was in. In spite of the DES debacle, the drug is still prescribed to, and used by, women for questionably effective purposes — for relieving breast engorgement or suppressing milk flow after they have a baby.

The female hormones, estrogen and progesterone, are also prescribed, ineffectively as it turns out, to prevent threatened abortions. The incidence of birth defects among children of women exposed to hormones during the first three months of pregnancy is from two to five times higher than the incidence among children whose mothers were not exposed to the drugs. The Food and Drug Administration withdrew approval of these drugs for use in pregnancy in December 1973 and in February 1974, but this ban did not seem to stop the use of them. In 1975, physicians wrote more than half a million prescriptions for the use of hormones during pregnancy.

Estrogen therapy is also a hotly disputed therapy for menopausal women. At first it seemed logical to replace the estrogens no longer supplied naturally by the body when menopause begins, but as menopausal women began taking estrogens, physicians started noting an increase in the incidence of cancer of the uterus. In 1977, the FDA ruled that the five million middle-aged women who take estrogens for a year or longer must be warned that they are multiplying, by a factor ranging from five to ten, the normal risk of cancer of the uterus.

"You may have heard that taking estrogens for long periods after the menopause will keep your skin soft and supple and keep you feeling young," warned a statement to the public from the FDA. "There is no evidence that this is so, however, and such long-term treatment carries important risks."

Estrogen therapy given to females at the other end of the life cycle — premenstrual — is also highly controversial. Estrogen treatment can cut several inches from a child's eventual height when taken in doses ten to 100 times stronger than birth control pills over a period of years.

During childhood, bone first appears as flexible cartilage, which grows with the child. Although doctors do not fully understand the chemistry of bone fusion, the female and male sex hormones that are secreted when puberty begins somehow hasten the final conversion of cartilage into bone, and growth stops. By the time their menstrual cycle begins, girls have completed 95 percent of their growth.

Inducing puberty in a nine-year-old girl — menstruation, breast development, growth of pubic hair — is a serious tampering with natural development. Is being a six-foot woman so disastrous that it is worth this tampering? Then, too, estrogens are poorly understood and are indicted as possible agents of breast and uterine cancer. Is being tall — or even very tall — worse than the risk of cancer?

Though estrogen treatments may be an effective way to control height in young girls, pediatric endocrinologists disagree on how safe it is. Several refuse to treat tall stature at all; others reserve treatment for cases in which the child and family seem sufficiently disturbed to justify the risks.

*

There is no end to the wonders of a modern cure. Researchers working with a cholesterol-lowering drug found that they can cut the incidence of heart attacks at the price of inducing gallbladder disease. But the gallbladder disease can be controlled by another drug. The side effects of the second drug are not yet known. Is it worth taking two drugs, one with known side effects, to counteract high cholesterol levels, when these levels can be lowered in many people by diet?

Cancer treatments also are notorious for their snowball effect: they treat disease as well as cause it. According to the Memorial Sloan-Kettering Cancer Center, 5 to 10 percent of cancer patients develop a second cancer, testimony to the fact that the lives of more and more cancer patients are being extended through chemotherapy and radiation long enough for a second cancer to develop. The second cancer sometimes is not merely due to the patient's living longer, but living long enough so that the cancer therapies have time to do their damage. A second cancer is now acknowledged to be a possible complication of cancer treatments. It is time to "examine the fine print in Faust's pact with the devil," said one cancer researcher. (The problems of personal decision-making about cancer treatments among the terminally ill are discussed in Chapter 9.)

*

The limits of medicine remain elusive, but hopes for a cure remain high. These hopes often blur realities, and in the endless pursuit of good health doctors and patients to-gether keep a silent compact as questions about safety, ap-propriate use, efficacy, and side effects go unasked.

Take a drug, go to the hospital for surgery, follow a certain diet. And all without a question from the patient or an explanation by the doctor. A retired schoolteacher, on the advice of an endocrinologist, took pills for more than two years to shrink a growth on her thyroid. The pills, however, affected the functioning of her thyroid, so she was prescribed two additional drugs to bring it back to normal. The second round of pills did their job well; they counteracted the effect of the thyroid-shrinking pill. But they really were not neces-sary. When the woman consulted with her long-time family physician, he told her, "You could take this pill until Christ-mas in the year two thousand and it still won't shrink this kind of growth you have." Yet she was on a potentially life-long regimen of three drugs per day — and none of them was needed. Who is to blame? The physician, for prescribing the drug? Or the limits of pharmacology?

"Patients don't want to offend their physician," Albert Jonsen explained. "They are somewhat dependent on their doctors and feel very grateful toward them. Patients also often feel foolish asking questions." If Sam Smith asks his doctor if a drug he just prescribed will do harm, the physician responds, "Of course it won't hurt; I gave it to help you." Should Smith question his doctor further? After all, Smith did come for help, and that is just what his doctor says he is giving. But think about all the DES mothers who took the drug because their physicians recommended it.

The classic model for a doctor-patient relationship is the Big Daddy model: the doctor tells the patient what to do. Patients are active partners in health-care decisions only in that they seek help and are willing to cooperate. After that, medical decisions are in the doctor's hands. This approach underlies most of medical practice, said Stuart Spicker, phi-losopher and bioethics teacher at the University of Connecti-cut Health Center. "You walk into the doctor's office with a complaint and you are guilty — diseased — until he proves you are innocent — healthy."

The doctor-patient relationship is changing as technological advances change the composition of health care. Physicians are refusing to do all that their patients request. Most doctors, for example, disapprove of parents aborting a fetus of the unwanted sex, and refuse to perform an amniocentesis for sex-determination purposes. Patients, too, are beginning to refuse treatments urged by physicians. Sloan Oliphant, the sixty-five-year-old man dying of cancer of the esophagus introduced in Chapter 1, made a conscious decision not to have any more radiation treatments for his unrelenting cancer.

Compassion in medicine is changing, wrote Barnard College sociologist Bernard Barber in the *New England Journal of Medicine*. "In the traditional pattern of doctor-patient relation, the appropriate form of compassion is paternalistic benevolence. It is the physician — active, decisive, individualistically responsible — who defines and dispenses compassionate care." In a newer pattern, Barber continued, compassion is expressed by actions the doctor takes that are socially meaningful to the patient.

A compassionate doctor in the old mold would have saved Sloan Oliphant's life at all costs, with more tests, more treatments. Following the new model, Oliphant's doctor made home visits and gave pain-relieving medicine — not attempts at "curing" terminal cancer — while Oliphant prepared to die at home, with his close family members talking to him by his bedside.

The need to be compassionate, to offer patients alternatives, becomes more imperative not only because of the underlying ethics, but also because of the fear of malpractice. Besides severe injury, the major cause of malpractice, according to HEW's Malpractice Commission, relates to the doctor-patient relationship: a breakdown of rapport between the doctor and patient; patients' frustration with the way complaints are handled; and unrealistic expectations by patients based on misinformation or lack of communication with the doctor.

"The medical marketplace is changing. Doctors will no longer have a God-like stature," said the Reverend David Duncombe, chaplain at Yale Medical School, "because people want the right to participate in vital decisions which affect their lives."

Chapter 6

Birth Pangs

THE SIGNS of imminent birth are clear: long powerful contractions of the uterus prepare for the separation of a baby from its mother's womb. As nature begins to run its normal course — and each contraction of the cervix slightly enlarges the opening to the womb to make room for the baby's passage — the medicalization of birth takes over. Drugs can induce labor or postpone it. Painkillers numb senses; anesthesia removes consciousness. Computers record fetal activity, and some surgeons barely wait for the first sign of distress before removing the baby from the womb.

Since most American babies are born normal, healthy, and without complications, is all this technology really necessary? Is pregnancy and its final stage — labor — a disease, a serious medical condition, or a natural state of development?

Monitoring the Beginning of Life

The latest in a long line of technological advances that have been accepted in common medical practice is the electronic fetal monitor, a machine that continuously records the fetal heartbeat in relation to contractions. The to-be-born baby is monitored either externally, with a belt of electrodes strapped to the mother's abdomen, or internally, with an electric lead shielded in a catheter inserted in the mother, making its way directly to the scalp of her baby.

The rationale behind fetal monitoring is that the condition of a fetus can deteriorate rapidly during the stress of labor, especially during long contractions, when oxygen supplies to the baby are cut off temporarily. So-called fetal distress can result in mental retardation as well as death, but if changes in the fetal heart rate are discovered by electronic monitors, a quick delivery by Caesarean section might save the lives of some of the 7500 babies who die each year in labor.

As a result of this new life-saving technology, many hospitals, particularly those in metropolitan areas, are using electronic fetal monitoring on every patient, or on as many as they have machines and personnel to service. Who wouldn't want to prevent death or irreversible brain damage? Who wouldn't want electronic monitoring?

The answer is not a simple one. Women do want to protect their baby from harm, but many prefer an alternative form of vigilance, which is less invasive. The external monitor severely limits a mother's mobility. She must be bed-bound and cannot turn freely from side to side. Internal monitors provide more freedom for the mother, but the price for this freedom is the highly invasive technique described above.

Listening, not watching, is an alternative way to monitor fetal movements — listening with an old-fashioned stethoscope. However, this method is less accurate than electronic monitoring, and even a careful nurse listens to fetal heartbeats with a stethoscope only every five to fifteen minutes.

Should all babies be electronically monitored? Who has the right answer?

("Start to use a fetal monitor with the first signs of labor," says Dr. Mary Kate Davitt, head of the neonatal intensive care unit at Georgetown University Hospital.

("Save it [fetal monitoring] for the high-risk pregnancies," advises Dr. Albert Haverkamp, obstetrician and gynecologist at the University of Colorado Medical Center. High-risk pregnancies include women who have a previous history of premature labors or babies dying in labor, those with high blood pressure, toxemia, and diabetes. A pregnancy is also high-risk if an abnormal heart rate is detected by use of the stethoscope.

₵"Every child should be monitored," says Dr. Frederick C. Green, associate director of the Children's Hospital in Washington, D.C. But Green questions whether this has to be done electronically. "My grandfather was a country doctor, and he knew how to listen."

Clinical studies have produced much conflicting data, and researchers have not yet proven the benefits of fetal monitoring. One study purported to show that failure to monitor high-risk groups increases the risk of fetal death by nearly two times. But when 500 high-risk babies about to be delivered at Denver General Hospital were randomly divided into two groups — some electronically monitored and some monitored with stethoscopes — researchers, headed by Haverkamp, found no differences in the outcomes of the infants. Death rates, serious sickness, and time spent in the hospital were all similar.

Evidence for continuing the evaluation of electronic fetal monitors surfaced recently when a medical statistician in Vermont noted a 30 percent decline over a five-year period in the death of newborns in hospitals that used electronic fetal monitoring. But in other parts of the state, where nurses and physicians listened to fetal heartbeats with traditional stethoscopes, the same statistician noted a similar decrease in death rates.

What is the reason for the decreased mortality rate among newborns in Vermont and elsewhere in the U.S.? Is it fetal monitoring, better prenatal care, better nutrition, or improved technology in the intensive care nursery? The answers are not clear, but a deep-seated belief in the good that technology can bring is in part responsible for the rising use of fetal monitoring — even though its efficacy is not well established.

There are, in addition, many serious technological problems associated with fetal monitoring. Perforations of the uterus as well as uterine infections can be caused by the catheter, and about 3 percent of the babies develop abscesses from the electrodes inserted in their scalps.

Perhaps the most important complication of fetal monitoring is the danger of surgery, directly associated with the marked increase in Caesarean sections. Nearly three times as many women who are electronically monitored have C-sections, as compared with those monitored by stethoscope. Nationwide, more than 10 percent of the deliveries are done by Caesarean section — a doubling in six years. This increase is due in large part to the continuous electronic monitoring of fetal heartbeat, which alerts physicians to possible abnormalities and allows them to reach readily for their scalpel.

In 90 percent of all labors, there is some deceleration of heart tone. It is not known when a deceleration of heartbeats means that the baby is lacking oxygen, that the baby will die or be brain-damaged from an extended contraction, or that the baby will withstand the contraction stress and live a normal healthy life. It is known, however, that rapidly falling heartbeats often correct themselves. Should a physician gamble that this will happen, or should a rush Caesarean delivery be made? Which gamble is greater?

In the study at Denver General, patients monitored by nurses had less deceleration of heartbeats and less fetal distress. Dr. Haverkamp questioned why. "Perhaps the nurses did not notice distress symptoms which would have been picked up routinely by the electronic monitor. Or perhaps it was more comforting [for the mother] to be attended by a person rather than a machine. With mobility limited and the woman in labor continuously hearing her baby's heartbeat being recorded, the fetal monitor can provoke anxiety.

"It costs a thousand dollars to have a baby in a hospital," Haverkamp added. "We should give women some compassion for that amount of money. To place the emphasis on sophisticated technology as a way of further depressing neonatal deaths — and not in social programs such as better prenatal care and nutrition — may be a mistake."

Paradoxically, the increasing use of fetal monitors comes at the same time as a consumer push for less medical intrusion at birth. More and more women are having natural deliveries, and even though more than 98 percent of the babies born in the U.S. are born in hospitals, home deliveries are on the rise.

The conflict between naturalness and safety of birth remains unresolved. But since most babies are born without trouble, the vigilance, intrusion, loss of autonomy, and high costs involved in electronic fetal monitoring are clearly not necessary. This evaluation, however, is made with hindsight. Who can determine which of the pregnant population — both high-risk and low-risk women — will have babies in trouble? A normal pregnancy can turn into a disaster in a minute if the baby sits on its own umbilical cord and shuts off the vital supply of oxygen, causing irreversible cerebral damage. Who will make the decision as to which women are monitored, which ones are not?

Babies in Trouble

"Please be patient — God hasn't finished me yet," reads a card affixed to the Isolette in a neonatal intensive care unit. The sign was placed there by the mother of a four-pound infant, struggling to become finished.

Every year, about five of every 100 babies are born ill and require specialized care the moment they leave their mother's wombs. Some of them have inherited genetic disorders that require medical attention. Many mongoloid babies, for example, are born with gastrointestinal obstructions that must be repaired if the baby is to survive. Some babies have birth defects, such as heart problems that call for surgery; jaundice, which may involve total blood transfusions; or infections that may be fatal. But most of the babies in trouble are born prematurely. Their lungs are not developed fully enough, and they cannot breathe properly by themselves. In the more than 2000 nurseries in U.S. hospitals, intensive care can help save 85 percent of these babies in trouble.

The present-day neonatal intensive care unit resembles a space capsule full of electronic monitors and life supports. Infants are wired both for survival and surveillance. They eat through tubes in their noses, navels, or veins in the head; they breathe through respirators; and they stay alive only because of these manmade connections. Monitors continuously record bodily functions — heartbeat, blood pressure, blood oxygen, urine. If respiratory difficulty increases — as it often does — a buzzer sounds, and within a minute someone is there to adjust the delivery of oxygen. Too little oxygen could cause brain damage; too much could cause blindness.

*

In the early 1970s, a baby weighing two pounds at birth had a 20 percent chance of surviving. Half the babies that size were surviving by the late seventies.

The advent of modern technology cannot alone explain the drop in mortality. Consider the early history of Baby McG., as related by his physician in a Canadian medical journal. Baby McG. was born more than forty years ago, two months premature and so tiny that his physician recalled, "I did not expect survival. This was by far the smallest living baby I had ever seen." Baby McG. was indeed small: he weighed fourteen ounces. There was no incubator for Baby McG., but the nurse bathed him in warm olive oil, wrapped him in cotton, and placed him in a basket in a warm oven. One year after the baby's birth, his physician wrote that baby McG. was developing normally and was in good physical and mental condition.

Baby McG. was an isolated case of good luck. Today there are a lot of Baby McGs. surviving. "There are pressures to diminish neonatal mortality, to save everybody," commented pediatric neurologist David McCullough, at Georgetown. "And we *can* save everyone, but what do we have? Anoxia and severe loss of oxygen to the brain? A variety of congenital anomalies and severely crippling mental and physical handicaps? Neonatal survival statistics which include these kinds of survivors do not impress me."

Is it worthwhile to use expensive sophisticated technologies to preserve life if the ultimate prognosis is so questionable? At the Los Angeles Cedar-Sinai Medical Center, the cost of caring for seventy-five premature babies was recently calculated. It was predictably high, even staggering. The total tab for each infant who died after an average of seventeen days was $14,126. For each survivor staying an average of three months, the cost soared to $40,287. The director of the intensive care nursery justified these costs when weighed against other expensive medical technologies: "Bypass procedures are generally done on many people who are nearing the end of their productive lives. In contrast, this group of patients is at the very beginning of life."

Until recently as many as 70 percent of the surviving low-birthweight babies had severe handicaps. But the prognosis for premature newborns is greatly improving, and the handicap rate has dropped to 5 to 15 percent. This includes only identifiable handicaps, such as mental and physical disabilities, not soft data, such as learning disabilities. Most neonatologists assume that many of the very low-birthweight survivors will have problems in school. "They will probably graduate from high school," predicted Dr. Davitt, "but college may be too demanding for them."

One of the reasons for the decrease in handicaps is a better understanding of the body's mechanisms. Predictive tests can pinpoint problems, and rational treatment can mitigate difficulties. But medical treatments in early life or even before birth are not without controversy. Treating immature lungs provides a good example.

Fetuses breathe not through their lungs but through an exchange of gases that pass through the placenta. Since they are not needed, the immature lungs are uninflated. But before birth, fetal lung begins to prepare for the instantaneous change from the fetus' dependence on the placenta to dependence on lungs. As part of this process, lung mucus is formed. Since it spills over into the amniotic fluid, a simple test of the fluid determines whether or not this mucus is present — indicating if the lungs are ready to take over the work of breathing or if respiratory problems are likely.

Steroids administered directly to the mother — and indirectly to the fetus — can mature lung capacity within one week. The results of this experimental treatment are encouraging as data accumulate and as the babies develop fewer and less serious kinds of respiratory distress.

But the full story is not yet in on treating fetuses with steroids. "If we can turn on one organ system and allow it to develop prematurely, perhaps we will inadvertently turn on another organ system. What additional unknown risks might there be?" asked Dr. John Berryman. Researchers already know that a growth stimulant for muscle and cartilage cells, a hormone that could be used one day to treat slow-growing fetuses with developmental defects, stimulates growth of cancer cells later in life.

"Steroids are being given," Berryman continued, "because we *believe* they do a lot of good, even though we do not know the long-term effects. Compounding the problem, how can we not offer it to someone when it might help her child?"

The ethical balance is a precarious one:

❬Let the infant struggle along in the neonatal intensive care unit for months at great financial cost, the risk of emotional damage, and a strong chance of mental retardation.

❬Let the infant die without taking advantage of any of the life supports in the intensive care unit.

❬Or give a twenty-eight-week-old fetus an experimental drug that provides the benefit of maturing the lungs but carries an unknown risk of unknown magnitude.

"We are talking about altering seventy years of a life," said Dr. Berryman. "Who decides whether to gamble on the unknown effects of a drug when the stakes are so high?"

*

The big question in neonatal care is how much care is too much, and when does it become extraordinary? When twenty-nine-year-old Linda Culbertson was critically injured in a traffic accident, she was rushed by medical helicopter to the nearest special emergency center. She had suffered head, neck, and internal injuries and was placed on a respirator. When she arrived at St. Anthony's Hospital, in Denver, the respirator registered no signs of brain activity. Her life-support system would normally have been disconnected at this point, based on the evidence of brain death. Instead, she was transferred to Colorado General Hospital, to serve as a possible organ-transplant donor.

It was at this time that physicians discovered that she was fifteen weeks pregnant, and the hospital staff decided to save her unborn baby. If they could keep Mrs. Culbertson alive for only five more weeks, the physicians felt they had a chance to deliver a viable baby of twenty weeks' gestation. "The decision was kind of automatic," reported a hospital spokesman. "When they detected another life, they decided to try to save it. What else could you do in a situation like that?"

Two days later, however, Mrs. Culbertson's doctors decided the case was medically hopeless and morally questionable, and her family agreed that she be allowed to die. The respirator was disconnected, and the mother and fetus immediately died.

A similar case happened in Brooklyn. Twenty-seven-year-old Rosemarie Maniscalo had mysteriously fallen into a coma, but she and her four-month-old fetus succumbed after a two-week attempt to save their lives. Mrs. Maniscalo was first thought to be brain-dead, but later her physicians reported that even though she had suffered severe brain damage, she still had minimal electrical brain activity. She died of a heart attack in spite of the respirator and the tube-feeding that was keeping her caloric intake high enough to maintain her and her fetus.

More cases like this will no doubt occur, and at least one attempt to save a small fetus will succeed. Fetuses substantially further along in development have been born to women in comas. A healthy six-and-a-half-pound girl was born re-

cently in Texas twenty-one days after her mother, Laurie Goforth, suffered two cardiac arrests, went into a coma, and was
placed on a life-support system. Mrs. Goforth was then thirty-
three weeks pregnant, and her doctors considered doing a
Caesarean section to get the fetus out but felt that, with the
extra trauma, it might die. They decided not to intervene with
the pregnancy and waited instead until Mrs. Goforth went
into natural labor. Their choice for life worked, but after the
birth, Mrs. Goforth, who had suffered irreversible brain damage, was weaned from the respirator so that she could die.

Where should the line be drawn? Forty percent of all con-
ceptions result in miscarriages, and about half of them are due
to chromosomal errors. This is nature's way of handling the
kinds of babies physicians call "gorks," because "God only
really knows" why they are born. As neonatal care becomes
better and better, should attempts be made to save the lives
of naturally aborted fetuses? If society decides that every baby
should be salvaged, who should provide funds and facilities to
meet their continuing medical and psychological needs? Is
this the responsibility of the parents? Of society?

Though it is perplexing to know how far to go in the use of
new life-saving alternatives, the more germane, ethically laden
question is whether the use of the technology is appropriate.
"In the case of extreme immaturity — say, a twenty-week baby
weighing eight hundred grams [1½ pounds], the ventilator
has nothing to offer to keep the baby alive. It only prolongs
the agony of dying," said Dr. John Raye, chief neonatologist
at the University of Connecticut Health Center. "We don't
think a baby like this will ever have the potential of breathing
independently. Using the ventilator in this case is showing off
the technology, and it is not appropriate."

Making Decisions for Appropriate Treatment

The technology is available to save — or at least to treat
heroically — every baby in trouble. Should every child be
saved? Yale pediatrician Raymond Duff blew the whistle in

1973 and reported in the *New England Journal of Medicine* that at the Yale–New Haven Hospital decisions are made to withhold treatment from very sick babies — babies with an extremely poor or even hopeless prognosis for a meaningful life.

The deaths of 14 percent of the babies, Duff revealed, were "associated with the discontinuance or withdrawal of treatment." The babies in this group were severely impaired by congenital disorders — chromosomal abnormalities, major heart defects, open spinal cords. Intensive efforts were made to save the lives of these babies, but at some point during the course of treatment, physicians, nurses, and parents realized the fight was hopeless, and they gave up after a period ranging from one day to five months.

There was less inclination to "give up" when the babies in trouble were very sick only because they were very little. If these babies could survive the traumas of their premature birth, went the reasoning, they could conceivably get better and lead normal lives.

Is normality a criterion on which to base a life-and-death medical decision? Are there degrees of normality that are more — or less — acceptable? Sociologist James R. Sorenson, interviewing families who had experienced the birth of a child with a genetic defect, found that the most acceptable genetic diseases are those that don't show. These are the kinds of conditions that impair physical functioning, but in a nonvisible way. Youngsters with diabetes, for example, look and act like normal healthy children except for dietary restrictions and lifelong dependency on insulin injections. Physical handicaps like blindness or deafness are more acceptable than impaired mental functions; a combination of the two plunges to the bottom of the scale of acceptability.

Take the controversial issue of Down's syndrome. About 25 percent of mongoloid children need surgery, most often to correct intestinal obstructions. Without the surgery, the surgery, the infants would probably die. Is this surgery extraordinary care? Should it be withheld? In a random sampling, 50 percent of the physicians in the San Francisco Bay Area polled by the University of California School of Public Health at Berkeley approved of withdrawing treatment for mongoloid babies with obstructions.

There is an awesome finality about making a decision to withhold treatment — to want a particular baby to die. The potential for error in prognosis makes the choice more agonizing for families and physicians. But the decision *not* to decide the merits of treatment or no treatment in a specific case is a decision by default.

Not every baby in trouble causes parents and doctors to undergo the ordeal of difficult decision-making. Only 10 percent of the babies in the neonatal ICU have problems which are so sticky that they require soul-searching decisions. "In most cases in the nursery there are not even the medical grounds for nontreatment. Difficult decisions are not provoked for every baby born with a congenital abnormality," Dr. Davitt said, "but they are raised when the quality of life is severely compromised.

*

Children born with spina bifida, a malformation of the central nervous system in which the spinal cord fails to develop correctly, provide a good example of the difficulties in making decisions about how to treat very sick babies. More than 12,-000 babies are born each year in the U.S. with this condition, and each case requires an agonizing decision.

Spina bifida is also called open-spine syndrome, because part of the spinal cord has little or no covering. It is exposed to the surface in the form of a large raised sac, which is often an oozing mass. The defect in the spinal cord also results in varying degrees of paralysis of the legs, bladder, and bowels. In more than 80 percent of the cases, excess spinal fluid collects in the head, causing hydrocephalus, which, if untreated, invariably results in mental retardation.

Fifteen years ago, 80 percent of the children born with spina bifida died; today, 80 percent live. The reason for this drastic change in the mortality rate is a policy, introduced by a group of physicians at the University of Sheffield, in England, of performing surgery immediately after birth. A shunt — an implanted system of tubing with a valve — is placed in the brain to drain excess fluid to another part of the body (usually the abdomen), where it is absorbed. The shunt eliminates head swelling and reduces the incidence of mental retardation. The opening in the spine is also closed as soon as the baby is born, thus reducing the risk of fatal infection.

As with all medical technology, success breeds popularity. Once the success of surgery for spina bifida was known, virtually all babies with the condition were treated aggressively. However, one of the Sheffield physicians who set out to save all spina bifida babies, Dr. John Lorber, soon realized that this approach might not be wise. "The indiscriminate use of advanced techniques of all types has kept alive those who should have died," he wrote in a British medical journal. "These babies now live with distressing physical or mental handicaps or both, often for many years, without hope of ever having an independent existence compatible with human dignity."

Lorber reviewed the records of 848 infants with spina bidida whom he had treated between 1959 and 1968. His findings were alarming. In spite of intensive care, operations, and advanced medical treatment, only 50 percent of the babies had survived. What concerned Lorber was the quality of life of the survivors: only 1.4 percent were normal — without any handicaps. All this effort — as many as eighteen operations in nine years for one young girl — and little more than 1 percent survived intact.

What about the rest of the survivors? More than 80 percent were severely physically handicapped, and almost half of this group were mentally retarded as well. The remaining 17 percent had moderate handicaps — lack of urinary control, which leads to frequent infections and renal failure; hydrocephalus, which must be continually controlled with shunts that have to be replaced as the child grows. And although most could walk with braces or move about in a wheelchair, they had deformities of spine, feet, and legs that required several operations to correct.

What kinds of lives were saved? "The problems we created were greater than those we solved," Lorber said. "Treating all babies, without selection, resulted in much more suffering for large numbers. Perhaps worst of all, because severely affected infants were 'saved,' many more potentially normal lives never started, because their parents did not dare to have children for fear of having a second child with spina bifida."

Given this predicament, some pediatric neurologists began evaluating critically which babies would benefit the most from the aggressive treatment, and came up with guidelines that indicate who will be good survivors. Early surgery is recommended if a baby has only one major problem: hydrocephalus, complete paraplegia, a spinal opening high on the back, or additional spinal defects. More than one of these defects usually indicates a low probability of survival or a poor quality of life.

*

How valid are these criteria? Can physicians really predict the extent of long-term disability at birth? Are physicians seers? The prognosis for Brian Barr was predicted a few hours after his birth. And Dr. David McCullough, in charge of the Spina Bifida Service at the Georgetown University Hospital, was precisely correct.

When Brian was born in the breech position, his mother, Marylou, immediately saw that something was wrong with his lower back. The doctor told the stunned Barrs about spina bifida. "Here they are, telling me about the second-highest birth defect, and I had never heard of it before," remembered Nick Barr, a physicist with the Defense Department.

McCullough was optimistic about Brian's chance for a good life. He did not have hydrocephalus, and his spine opening was low, so the paralysis was minimal. Brian had leg deformities — one foot was clubbed, the other bent back toward his leg — but these could be corrected with surgery.

"McCullough's descriptions of what would happen to Brian were encouraging," said Marylou Barr. "You hear that there's a problem with the spine and you think the worst. I thought he would be totally paralyzed, but Dr. McCullough said that there was a good chance Brian would walk."

The Barrs trusted McCullough's recommendation to operate, although it did cross Nick's mind that maybe they should forget it, and Marylou secretly wished that Brian had been born dead. Ten hours after he was born, Brian had his first and most important life-saving operation: his spinal opening was closed.

The Barrs have had their problems in bringing up a child with handicaps. Brian is only five and has had several operations on his feet; he bruises himself often because of the awkward way he walks ("in a flatfooted position like a clown," as his mother described it); and he once spent six weeks in a full-body cast when the doctors were trying to heal external ulcers from the bruises. Most bothersome is his incontinency — lack of bowel and urine control — which will be a lifelong problem.

"But Brian is an Aries," said Marylou, "a real ram, very strong-willed. He is very bright, very articulate, and his future looks good."

*

Dr. McCullough predicted a good outcome for Brian based on criteria present at birth. But he is not as optimistic about most of the babies he sees. At Georgetown, about 20 percent of the spina bifida babies are given such a poor prognosis that they are not treated. "We make them warm and comfortable, we feed them and love them," said Kathleen Quinn, nurse and coordinator of the Spina Bifida Service, "but we do not do any surgery and we do not treat infections. We are the ones who give the parents the idea of negative treatment, but they have to make the decision whether to accept or reject the proposal. Most of the parents accept it."

The LaFontaines accepted this alternative and knew from the day that their son, Adam, was born that he would die within a few months because they decided not to treat him. Joan LaFontaine had had two miscarriages before she conceived Adam, and she was naturally anxious about her third pregnancy. She suspected that something was wrong because she could feel the baby moving in only one place. The reason soon became clear: Adam was paralyzed from the chest down, so only his arms moved.

Adam was born with a severe case of spina bifida. His spinal cord had a large and seeping sac, he had a serious curvature of the spine, and though he did not have hydrocephalus at birth, he developed it shortly after.

"Before I realized that there would be any decision for me to make," recalled Joan, "he was rushed to the Georgetown nursery immediately after his birth. I had already signed a consent form allowing surgery to be performed on him. The hospital could have done the surgery, but they didn't. Because they didn't do the operation on his back immediately, I began to think that maybe it was more serious than we thought. Maybe nothing could be done."

Dr. McCullough and Kathleen Quinn explained the situation to the LaFontaines. They said that Adam's life expectancy with treatment was not known, but it was not likely that he would outlive adolescence. They described all the operations he would need just to stay alive, but pointed out that the benefits from them would be minimal. McCullough and Quinn also raised the idea that, in similar cases, some people choose a nontreatment route.

While lying in her hospital bed, Joan tried to make up her mind what to do. "Adam's life would be so bleak. He would never have any time just to be a normal child. The operations didn't seem to get to the core of things. He would still not be able to enjoy life. I decided not to treat him."

Her husband, Norman, independently came to the same conclusion.

The LaFontaines — Adam, Joan, and Norman — were together for a brief four months. "The quality of many years of suffering would not be as good as the quality of the few months we had together," Joan LaFontaine said. "Having these thoughts was the only way I could live with my decision."

From that day on, Adam received only passive nursing care. When his back leaked, his parents put on a sterile gauze pad. When he was nearly four months old, the sac burst open, and that proved to be a turning point. "After that, Adam never smiled, never followed us with his eyes or played with his mobile. We really lost him then," said Joan. A week later, he developed breathing problems and became lethargic, and when he was four and a half months old, Adam died of pneumonia.

Joan looks back philosophically at this bleak period of her life. "I fulfilled my moral responsibility to Adam. I made my child's life as full as possible, gave him a life of awareness, one in which he fulfilled his potential. If I had given him a prolonged life as a vegetable, I would not have been as responsible a parent. But," she added, "we really will never know how he would have responded to all of the operations. I see the moral dilemma of not treating, but I am still comfortable with our decision.

"I don't feel guilty — just sad for our little boy, who could never run and play and enjoy the sun. We loved him so much," she said softly.

*

The Barrs and the LaFontaines were fortunate, in spite of their hardships. The parents were given a correct prognosis of their child's outcome and could prepare for it accordingly. The Holtons were not so lucky. When Theresa was born, she had a large opening in her spine, hydrocephalus, a deformed spine, and was paralyzed from the chest down. She was not expected to survive the night, and the physicians recommended that she not be treated. Her parents, Phyllis and Van, agreed.

"Why prolong life?" questioned Phyllis. "The doctors told us she would die, and you believe what doctors tell you even though you know that they're not God and can't be sure. But," Phyllis added bitterly, "if they weren't so sure, they shouldn't have told us that Theresa was going to die — because she didn't."

Theresa tenaciously hung on to life for a full year before she received any life-saving treatment. Her head was already substantially enlarged from hydrocephalus when a shunt was implanted — a procedure the state institution required if she was to become a patient there. A partially treated youngster like Theresa is less likely to die than someone with no treatment, but she was still at risk for spinal fluid loss and fatal infections unless the opening on her back was repaired. The lesion on her back was subsequently closed.

Theresa is now five years old — sickly, plagued with convulsions and respiratory problems, including pneumonia. She is physically stunted and mentally retarded. "Van and I put her through a lot by making the decision not to operate when she was first born," Phyllis said, "but we thought it was the best thing to do. We were told her life would be over soon."

A Family Ordeal

There is no universal way that life-and-death decisions are made in the nursery. Some hospitals have guidelines; some have ethics committees; some leave the decision to the parents; in others, the physicians are in charge.

One young pediatrician felt very strongly about saving a particular baby in severe respiratory distress, and convinced the parents to agree to his using all the heroic measures available. He achieved his goal, but the infant survived only as a vegetable — a flaccid boy with little motor control and negligible mental function. At whose expense did that pediatrician practice his ethics?

Is an ethics committee in any better position to make the decision? Most hospitals have what are popularly called God Committees — a selected group of physicians, health professionals, and religious, legal, and ethics experts who decide the merits of a particular case. "Do they decide or do they pontif-

icate?" Raymond Duff asked in his Yale Medical School office.
"Members of the ethics committee are distant from the lives
of the people involved. As a result, they don't feel the heat
the way those living with the decision do."

Accordingly, the family should make the decision. But can
parents suffering from the shock of the birth of a defective
child make an ethical decision concerning treatment? "From
years of dealing with families, I believe that those who share
decision-making generally understand the issues well, make
difficult choices as well as anyone else and often better," said
Duff. "Not all families will decide prudently. But will a committee be more satisfactory? They don't have to live with the
consequences so they can ignore them."

*

The ordeal of Sally and Bill Brown, an attractive couple in
their late twenties, illustrates many of the problems encoun-
tered in making decisions about treating and not treating very
sick babies. In spite of the conflicting medical opinions about
virtually everything concerning the Browns' case — including
the prognosis of their son's life span — a decision had to be
made. Postponement could have meant death by default.

The Browns had been married for five years, and were looking forward to a family, when Jason, their first child, was born.
"I knew something was wrong," Sally said, recalling those early
confused moments after Jason's birth, "because the nurse put
him on the other side of the room and gave the doctor a note.
I thought maybe a finger was missing, or that he had a birth-
mark."

Either would have been a minimal problem compared with
what actually was wrong. The doctor took Bill aside and told
him that the baby looked suspiciously like a mongoloid. His
features were not as prominent as in other children with
Down's syndrome, so the doctor could not be sure until the
results of chromosomal tests became available in a few days.

"Jason's being retarded bothered me," said Sally, "but we
still loved him and wanted him very much. He was a healthy

baby, and we were looking forward to going home together — no matter what the results of the test."

What also bothered Sally was not knowing. The obstetrician thought Jason had Down's syndrome, but the pediatrician thought there was a 90 percent chance that nothing was wrong.

When Jason was a few days old, the Browns' world started to fall apart. On Wednesday, the final word came that Jason did have Down's syndrome. On Thursday, he developed a feeding problem. On Friday, he turned blue and began throwing up violently. X-rays showed a virtually complete blockage in his upper intestine, a situation that required immediate surgery.

The Browns agreed that surgery should be performed — in fact, they never questioned that it *not* be done — and they had him transferred to Georgetown University Hospital's neonatal intensive care unit. Again they were confronted with conflicting information. The neonatologist said that surgery could alleviate the problem; the pediatric surgeon felt that surgery could be done but recommended against it; and their private pediatrician said he wasn't sure if surgery could help but that with this type of mental retardation maybe it was better to let nature take its course.

Treating — or not treating — mongoloid children is a poorly understood issue, because mental retardation is not a sufficient reason for an infant not to live. "The decision to treat a baby with a birth defect depends on the severity of the malformation — not on whether the child is mentally retarded," explained Dr. Davitt in the Georgetown special nursery. "Doing open-heart surgery on a Down's syndrome baby is less controversial than doing surgery on the duodenum [upper intestine], because a heart operation is a dangerous procedure that has a lot of morbidity associated with it. The ethics issue is raised over the degree or gradation of difficulty of the procedure."

Whom should the Browns have believed? What should they have done — request the surgery or withhold treatment?

The Browns were in a no-win situation. "No matter which way we went," Bill said, "we would always question our decision. If Jason had the surgery and lived a difficult life, we would blame ourselves. If he died within a few days, we would blame ourselves."

Sally and Bill consulted with their family priest, who assured them that there would be no moral complication with the Catholic Church, no matter what they decided. Sunday — a week after Jason's birth — Bill made his decision after he asked himself probing questions: What if it were me? Would I want to spend a life like that? It's all right as a child, but what about when he's a teen-ager or an adult? If he became aware of his retardation, would that hurt him? Bill's answers led to one conclusion: no surgery.

Sally, too, tried to put herself in Jason's place. "There was no way I wanted to grow up like that," she said, as she agreed not to have the surgery.

The Browns informed the hospital of their decision, but Dr. Davitt asked them to reconsider it at a later day. "It was as if she was trying to talk us out of our decision," Sally recalled angrily. "She didn't know what we went through to make that decision." Davitt was not trying to have them change their mind, but, rather, she wanted to make sure that the Browns were 100 percent certain about their decision.

The Browns reconsidered, but they stuck with their decision: no surgery for Jason.

Dr. Davitt outlined the program the hospital staff would follow. They would feed Jason normally, trying to get food past the blockage in his duodenum, but there would be no supplemental nutrition by intravenous feeding. Davitt predicted that Jason would dehydrate, lose weight, and die within seven to ten days.

The day after Davitt's prognosis, Sally and Bill came to visit Jason in the hospital. "As we walked into the nursery," Sally related, "conversation stopped. The nurses stared at us with resentment and with anger. They were trained to save lives, and they couldn't do anything for Jason because of our decision."

When Sally fed Jason, she was reminded again of the impact of her decision. "Here I was," she remembered, "a young mother feeding my baby who was throwing up, not getting enough nourishment, simply because of a decision we'd made. I talked to him and told him that the decision had been made out of love."

The staff of the ICU began to rebel. Many physicians and nurses disagreed with the Browns' decision. An ethicist was called in to discuss the issue, but he only raised more unanswerable questions. The staff finally requested that the hospital ethics committee review the case.

"At Georgetown, the ethics committee makes sure that the decision-making process for no-treatment conditions is not being abused or treated too lightly," explained Davitt. "We cannot consult a committee every time we want to turn off the respirator."

The committee — which included the medical director, various department chairmen, a social worker, the attorney for the hospital, and the chaplain — represented a broad spectrum of the hospital's interests. The committee felt that the Browns' approach was ethically appropriate. But this was a consensus decision, not a unanimous one. The dissenters, protecting the rights of the defective child, wanted the hospital to intervene and take the Browns to court on a child-abuse charge.

Bill Brown was furious when he heard about the ethics committee meeting. "This was my business, not theirs," he said a year later, still angry about the intrusion into his affairs.

Meanwhile, Jason was taking the matter into his own hands. He initially became dehydrated and lost weight, as Dr. Davitt had predicted. But then his weight loss stabilized, and soon he began gaining weight. The food somehow was getting past a barely visible pinpoint hole in the obstruction and was nourishing Jason — letting him live.

When life supports are withdrawn and a baby survives in spite of the lack of treatment, physicians call it "passing the trial of life." Jason was nearly three weeks old when he passed the test, and Dr. Davitt told the Browns that it could take a few weeks, even a few months, before he failed it.

Based on this new prognosis, the Browns changed their mind about not treating Jason. "Even though we'd made the right decision before — not to treat — now things were different, and we had to make another decision based on the new information," said Bill.

Bill decided first again: "To go ahead with the surgery so Jason can be corrected and come home. We'll give him the best life he can hope for." Sally concurred. "My second decision was like the first, it was made out of love for Jason. To let him lie there in the hospital for weeks and weeks, even months, was inhuman."

Jason is now a toddler, running around the Browns' apartment. Bill still feels the crushing blow of not having a normal child, but he and Sally are working hard to help Jason develop as best he can.

The Browns regret neither of their decisions. "A decision about life is a very personal one," Bill explained. "I don't think the law should make decisions for the parents, nor do I think the medical profession should make the decision. We have to live with the problem, and we can't put it on someone else's shoulders."

*

Who is ultimately responsible? Parents may decide not to treat an infant with extreme defects, but they may also decide not to treat an infant with minor defects. Who decides which defects are acceptable — the parents who live with the decision, or the physician who gives the medical orders? If a baby dies because less than heroic treatment was given, can the parents or physician be charged with neglect or homicide?

Bringing the problem into the open — talking, thinking, writing about it — is an important first step toward finding solutions to the ethics problems raised in the nurseries. "What we are doing is acknowledging that we have a great deal of control over living and dying," Dr. Raymond Duff made clear. "The question is not whether to use that control, but how to use it prudently."

Another way to resolve some of the burning issues raised in the nurseries is to prevent birth defects. Thousands of low-weight premature infants could develop into full-term healthy babies with better nutrition programs, better prenatal health care. And countless genetic mishaps could be detected and the babies' births averted through prenatal-detection programs. A prenatal blood test, for example, can determine whether fetal proteins are being shed from an open spine into the mother's blood — an indication of spina bifida. Physicians are beginning to screen pregnant women for elevated protein levels, and a blood test to check for spina bifida is likely to become a standard part of prenatal care.

With medical interventions before birth, during birth, and in the nursery, physicians are seeking to create better and healthier babies. The medical decisions involved in each intervention are heavily laden with ethical and legal implications. Making these decisions is popularly called playing God, but someone human must make each decision.

Chapter 7

Tools for Diagnosing

SHOSHANNA ABELES is an attractive, bright teen-ager — inquisitive about life, eager for new experiences, and thankful to be alive after a close brush with death. The latest and most controversial of medical technology's tools — the computerized axial tomographic (CAT) scanner — correctly diagnosed her ailment, which, if gone untreated, would have killed her.

The CAT gives information sooner, more precisely, and with less pain than other techniques. But it is controversial because it is a costly diagnostic device that does little to improve the overall health picture. The list of controversial diagnostic tools is an expanding one, as new devices to learn more about the inner workings of the body are developed. Adding to the confusion, the range of appropriate uses of diagnostic tools is vast and not clearly defined. As a result, there is much misinformation as well as misuse of the very technologies that can save lives.

The CAT Caper

When Shoshanna Abeles started fifth grade in the fall of 1973 in rural Frederick, Maryland, everything seemed wrong. She had a bad case of the flu, which was treated with antibiotics. As soon as she recovered from that, one of her eyes became so swollen that she could not open it. Probably a piece of hay from the barn infected it, thought her physician, and she was again treated with antibiotics.

In addition to her medical problems, Shoshanna was having other problems. She became so irritable and querulous that her teacher requested that Shoshanna be transfered to another class. Her parents assumed that this was part of her rebellious growing-up period and hoped her normal sweet disposition would soon return.

One evening, just before Hallowe'en, Shoshanna went upstairs to get ready for bed. She had just finished arguing with her mother when she went into convulsions, holding her body rigid, staring ahead with fully dilated pupils.

The picture was clearer now: her odd behavior was due to some problem in her brain, not to pre-teen antics. A more precise diagnosis was needed, and Shoshanna was to have several procedures performed before the source of her problem was uncovered.

A spinal tap indicated that she did not have meningitis, and head x-rays showed nothing abnormal. But an electroencephalogram, which is a record of the electric activity of the brain, showed brain-wave irregularities, and an arteriogram, which indicates the condition of the arteries that supply blood to the brain, revealed a large but unidentifiable mass.

Acting on a hunch, Shoshanna's pediatrician associated her convulsions and odd behavior with a brain abscess, though he could not confirm it with the diagnostic tools he had in the community hospital. He decided to put her on massive doses of antibiotics, on the theory that if he was right and it was an abscess, the drugs would help. If Shoshanna had a brain tumor, the drugs would not help — but they also would not harm.

But he still had to know exactly what the mass was in Shoshanna's brain. The traditional way of diagnosing brain growths at the time was a painful, dangerous, and very invasive procedure called pneumoencephalography, in which air blown into the brain cavities outlines the convoluted tissues on an x-ray plate.

"We were very irrational about what to do," recalled Shoshanna's mother, Ann Abeles, a member of the Biological
Sciences Faculty at Frederick Community College. "We had
to find out what the mass was; but did she have to undergo
the pain and danger of having air blown into her brain?" Mrs.
Abeles discussed her concern with a cousin, a physician practicing at the George Washington University Medical Center.
He suggested that a CAT scanner be tried.

This is how Shoshanna came to have her brain abscess diagnosed by the sophisticated, controversial CAT scanner. Physicians found and removed a tennis ball–sized abscess lodged
over her right eyebrow. Her pediatrician's hunch to treat her
with antibiotics — and her previous ailments, which had required them — turned out to be fortunate.

Physicians are still unclear about the cause of the abscess,
but Shoshanna has very definite opinions about their treatment of it. "Without the scanner, I'd be dead."

*

Shoshanna's tale illustrates medical diagnostic technology at
its best: it was used effectively, efficiently, and it saved the life
of a ten-year-old in trouble. The CAT scanner, developed in
England in the late 1960s and first used in 1970, has been
hailed as the greatest advance in radiology since the field was
created by the discovery of x-rays in 1895. It combines sophisticated x-ray equipment, which directs beams into the body
from nearly 300 different angles (the machine shifts 1° with
each scan), with a computer, which analyzes the information
and visually reconstructs cross sections of the insides of a body.
Tomography is from a Greek word meaning "to write a slice,"
and the computerized axial tomographic scanner does just
that: it records a detailed description of what a thin slice of
the patient looks like.

While the scanner is not a unique radiological tool — it
rarely uncovers things that were previously entirely hidden
from radiologists — it does see things in a relatively painless,
harmless way. Although it exposes people to radiation, it does

so at greatly reduced levels, when compared with traditional methods. When Shoshanna had the arteriogram, she was exposed to more than 10 rads (a rad is a standard measure of radiation exposure), and the cause of her problem was still not detected. The CAT, in contrast, not only detected the abscess but did so by adding relatively few rads to her total radiation exposure. An average series of head scans adds between 1 and 4.5 rads.

The CAT also replaces other painful and invasive diagnostic procedures. In a three-year study at George Washington, analyzing data on procedures performed before and after the installation of a head scanner, physicians found an 80 percent decrease in the use of pneumoencephalography, the painful and dangerous procedure that Shoshanna was scheduled to undergo but which her mother Ann questioned.

The only invasive feature of the scanner is the injection of dye, to show contrasts in the body — a procedure followed in about two thirds of the brain scans. While it is not painful, it is invasive. "The invasiveness is not only putting in the needle," said David Davis, neuroradiologist and associate chairman of the Department of Radiology at George Washington, "but also the ten ounces of contrast material running through a person. It can cause a rash or hives, and it does present a greater risk than using no contrasting color. But," he added, "it is also often necessary." Shoshanna's first scan indicated only that there was a mass in her brain. But after she was injected with an opaque dye, Davis discovered the special attributes of the mass that indicated it was an abscess.

In spite of the praises for the CAT scanner, it is the favorite whipping boy of health-care critics. It is big, expensive, overused, and overrated. One of the key controversial, and unanswered, questions is who should be scanned: every patient with a headache — and there are twelve million of them making visits to their physicians' offices each year — or only those with headaches plus a neurological problem, such as a seizure, blurred vision, weakness in one arm or leg?

"From a societal viewpoint, we could dump doing scans

for just headaches," Dr. Davis said, "since we see lesions in only less than one percent of the cases where headaches are the only complaint. But maybe we would be doing something good for these people [with headaches only] by doing the scan, and then they wouldn't have to worry anymore about having a brain tumor. They might be more useful to society this way."

There is no easy answer to the question of who should be scanned. "You can put everyone who needs an artificial kidney on dialysis because you can draw a line between those who have kidney failure and those who don't. But you can't draw such a fine line between those who need a scan and those who don't," cautioned internist H. David Banta, HEW health-care analyst and author of several reports raising questions about the scanner.

Among those people scanned, fully half get negative reports; that is, nothing wrong is found. Dr. Davis explained, "A negative scan is more important than a positive one because we can say with a high degree of accuracy — ninety-nine point five percent — that a person does not have something wrong. It helps the worried well — the thirty-five-year-old woman with headaches who worries about having a brain tumor."

What about the worried sick? If the CAT finds a tumor, often there is little that physicians can do to change the course of the disease. A pancreatic scan, for example, is not routinely performed until a patient shows symptoms of a cancer. By then, the scan is likely to uncover tumors in the pancreas that are large or have spread to other organs. Surgery, even radiation, is unlikely to save such patients.

The fine pinpointing of an incurable condition raises many moral dilemmas about health care. The right hemisphere of the brain, for example, is the center of emotions and judgment. Would it be morally acceptable to remove a part of the right side of the brain if the CAT discovers a tumor there? Is it more acceptable to remove part of the left side, which affects motor movement and speech?

Gay Kroeger, a former foreign service officer and mother of two young daughters, chose not to have an operation on the left side of her brain after the CAT detected a malignant brain tumor. The scan showed precisely where the tumor was, but neurosurgeons could also precisely predict a loss of 90 percent of her speech ability as well as loss of all movement on her right side.

Gay was given a diagnosis and a death sentence. Surgery — and the incapacitated life that would result from it — was unacceptable to both Gay and her husband, Arthur. She gambled instead on a full dose of cobalt treatment, in the hope of gaining three to six months of a good life. She suffered radiation burns, baldness, nausea, and loss of appetite, and was put on a strict regimen of twenty pills a day. But this course of treatment shrank the tumor and gave Gay an extra four years of good life — before her tumor reappeared.

As bad as the diagnosis was for Gay, at least it put an end to two years of unexplained seizures, as many as three a week. "I resented being told that I was a neurotic lady," Gay said, "and I was glad to know — finally — what was wrong with me, even if it is incurable."

Not all CAT scan diagnoses are without cures. Think of Shoshanna Abeles, or eighteen-month-old Michael Halloran, a red-haired boy whose parents were concerned because he seemed slow in passing such normal developmental milestones as crawling and standing. Michael's skull x-rays were normal, but a CAT scan showed that he had advanced hydrocephalus. A shunt was put in to drain the excess fluid that was accumulating in his brain, and because he was treated at a relatively young age, there is a good chance that he will develop as a normal child.

When thirty children from the St. Elizabeth's Home, a school for the educable and trainable retarded in West Philadelphia, were scanned, fully 30 percent were found to have tumors, cysts, excess fluid, or congenital malformations causing their mental problems. As with Michael, in several cases surgical procedures could have eliminated or substantially reduced mental retardation. But the scanner's diagnoses came too late to help most of the St. Elizabeth's children. "Every hospital with a patient load of over a hundred patients should have a brain scanner," said the radiologist who scanned the youngsters at St. Elizabeth's.

*

Not everyone agrees. "There is a CAT fever," wrote Harvard Medical School professors Stuart Shapiro and Stanley Wyman in the *New England Journal of Medicine,* and its symptoms are the "feverish impulse to own, operate, exploit or write about CATs. It has reached epidemic proportions and continues to spread among physicians, manufacturers, entrepreneurs and regulatory agencies."

The reason for the concern about CAT fever is the wild spread of a new technology before it is known for what purposes it is best used, how many of the instruments are needed, and where. The issue is not whether the scanner is a valuable diagnostic tool. Everyone agrees that it is. Shoshanna Abeles, Gay Kroeger, and Michael Halloran's stories testify to the ways treatment can be tailored specifically to an individual case once the details of the inner body are recorded by the scanner.

The issue is whether all of the machines in operation and on order are needed. By 1980 there will be 2500 scanners in operation in the U.S. Since each scanner costs from $350,000 to $700,000, that means an expenditure of more than $1 billion for one diagnostic device. A big investment, yes, but, with the great deal of use they get, the machines will rapidly pay for themselves: health planners anticipate $1 billion *annually* in CAT scan billings.

Are all these machines really necessary? Is supply creating the demand? In Washington, D.C., alone there are nearly two dozen head and body scanners. There are more scanners in use in southern California than there are in Great Britain, the birthplace of the scanner.

"Excesses [of the CAT] should be eliminated," asserted Dr. William Knaus, a Robert Wood Johnson Foundation Clinical Scholar at George Washington, "but not the CAT.

We should not keep it from anyone in the U.S. who can use it when and if the chance comes up that they need to be scanned."

Where, then, should scanners be placed? If everywhere is too much, how can selective placing of scanners be done equitably? Shoshanna was a patient in two small community hospitals before she was rushed by ambulance to the CAT scanner in Washington, one hour away. "If there had been a scanner here in Frederick, the course of Shoshanna's illness would have been less traumatic and disruptive for us," said Ann Abeles. "We would have known right away that she had an abscess and would not have thought she had a tumor. When the arteriogram showed a mass, we did worry — as it turns out, without need — that she had a tumor." Although Ann Abeles would have had less anguish if her local hospital had a scanner, she does not feel that every hospital, even every locality, needs one.

Controls are being instituted to stop CAT fever. A certificate of need (CON), according to federal statutes, must be granted by state and federal local health-planning agencies for any capital expenditure over $150,000 made by hospitals. The concepts of CONs — for scanners as well as other costly hospital equipment — has met with varying degrees of success. Hundreds of applications to purchase scanners have already been denied, at least temporarily. But when determined hospitals are barred from purchasing a scanner because they cannot prove a need, ingenious alternatives often emerge.

Consider what happened recently in Maryland. The state health planners allocated two CATs each to a few teaching hospitals in Baltimore but none in Annapolis, a half-hour drive away. Since hospitals but not private physicians have to have a certificate of need, a group of physicians banded together, purchased a machine, and leased space from an Annapolis hospital. They now have the machine they want — in the place they want it — in spite of CON regulations. A growing number of scanners — nearly 20 percent of the total — are purchased by similar groups of physicians.

"The major reason why hospitals or private physicians buy — or want to buy — the new technology is economics: they can make money from it," says a health-care critic. Why not put restraints on the money that can be made? The Institute of Medicine took a step in this direction in a 1977 report that recommended that third-party payers reimburse for CAT scanning services provided only by installations approved under a CON program. (The clout of third-party payers in controlling the spread of medical technology is discussed in Chapter 12.)

The chief lesson to be learned from the CAT caper is that new technology should be evaluated before it is bought. Dr. David A. Hamburg, president of the Institute of Medicine, said, "The concern about the CAT centers on the fact that it was bought on its promise rather than its proven capabilities."

The Mammography Muddle

It seemed like a sound idea when, in 1974, the National Cancer Institute, in collaboration with the American Cancer Society, set up the free Breast Cancer Demonstration Projects for women over thirty-five years of age. Statistics on breast cancer instill fear: 7 percent of American women — one out of fourteen — will develop it during their lifetime, and each year 88,000 new cases are diagnosed and 33,000 women die from it.

The screening program was an ideal chance to get at the breast cancer before it gets at you. The value of an early diagnosis is indisputable. When the cancer is detected and treated when the tumor is still confined to the breast, 84 percent of the women survive at least five years. But if the cancer goes undetected and spreads to the lymph nodes, the chances for survival are less favorable: only 55 percent of the women with advanced breast cancer will live longer than five years.

The climate was ripe for a program in early detection of

breast cancer. The first and second ladies of the country —
Betty Ford and Happy Rockefeller — both underwent surgery
for breast cancer. After their operations, there was a four- to
tenfold increase in requests for examinations in one of the
twenty-seven centers in the National Cancer Institute–American Cancer Society (NCI–ACS) breast cancer detection
program. A total of 280,000 women voluntarily came to have
their breasts x-rayed and manually examined once a year for
five years.

For all its good intentions, the mammography muddle
turned out to be similar to the CAT caper: hundreds of
thousands of people jumped on a bandwagon to use a diagnostic technology before its safety and efficacy were firmly
established.

The rationale for the screening program was an earlier
project, conducted in the 1960s by New York's Health Insurance Plan (HIP), which demonstrated that periodic
screening with mammography and physical examinations reduced breast cancer mortality in a group of 31,000 women
between the ages of forty and sixty-four. Over a nine-year
period, there were ninety deaths from breast cancer in the
group of women receiving mammographs, in contrast to 128
deaths in a similar group of women who did not have the
x-ray. The breast cancer death rate, according to the HIP
data, could be lowered by one-third if cancers were diagnosed
and treated at an earlier stage.

There were some caveats to the HIP study. Women under
fifty who had the x-rays had the same breast cancer death
rate as women who did not have the annual examination.
The benefits of screening, researchers concluded, were proven
only for women over fifty years of age. Nonetheless, the
NCI–ACS program enrolled women as young as thirty-five,
in spite of a warning from consultants to the project that
giving a woman under the age of fifty a mammograph on a
routine basis is "close to unethical."

The ethics issue concerned the risk of excessive radiation
exposure. "Radiation risk from one exposure doesn't show up

for five to ten years," said John C. Bailar III, the physician-statistician who is editor-in-chief of the *Journal of the National Cancer Institute* and one of the principal critics of the screening program. "A seventy-five-year-old woman who receives a breast x-ray is not likely to live on to that period of latency. But a woman who is thirty-five could live for forty more years, well into the latency period. Since younger women are likely to have more mammographies — they are scheduled to have one a year for five years in the detection program — they are at even greater risk."

It is also known that mammography will never be as effective in younger women as it is in older women because of the nature of women's breasts. Breast cells are dense in younger women, and it is difficult for x-rays to penetrate them. As women age, their cells become less dense, and it is easier for the x-rays to detect abnormalities.

"Mammography is not innocuous," Bailar cautioned. "Women must consider the risks as well as the benefits. The overall benefits of mammography in screening the general population have not been determined, and its hazards may be greater than are commonly understood. This marvelous technological gadget is used to attract women in for breast examinations which can also be done by nontechnological means."

During the summer of 1976 — two years after the 280,000 women flocked to the detection centers — they began staying away in droves. Fear of cancer was rampant again, but this time it was fear of getting cancer from the very machine that was to detect it. Newspaper articles warned women under fifty about the increased risks of getting cancer from the x-ray. NCI–ACS officials initially denied any risks; then, in an about-face move that helped further confuse the public, they issued guidelines recommending routine mammographies only for women over fifty.

Meanwhile, more than a quarter of a million women were caught in the middle of a battle between the pro- and anti-mammography groups. There was a 10 to 40 percent drop in women coming to the detection centers, and an unknown potential increase in breast cancer deaths as a result. The information about the radiation hazards raised such fears and confusion that at one major center, half of the dropouts were under fifty years of age, but half were over fifty — the very group the detection program aids.

Physicians, too, were confused and gave women conflicting opinions. One forty-four-year-old woman with no history of breast cancer in the family and no unusual breast problems requested a mammography simply because her physician recommended it. Contrast her to a thirty-eight-year-old woman who had a history of cystic breasts and previously had had two mammographies that showed abnormalities. She told the nurse at the detection center that her surgeon did not want her to have a mammography because "it might be too dangerous."

"Many women are very confused about whether to have a mammography or not, and they want us to make the decision for them," said Kathleen Foster, a nurse in an NCI–ACS breast cancer detection center. "For so many years, people did what the doctors said without questioning it. Now people are making decisions about their own bodies, and they are faced with the problem of not knowing what to do."

What is a risk worth? "Breast cancer occurs in one in fourteen women," commented Bailar, "but no one is recommending a prophylactic mastectomy for every woman. A one-in-fourteen risk is not great enough for that. But a one-in-one risk is. Where does the change occur between one in one and one in fourteen? Is one in four enough of a risk to warrant a prophylactic mastectomy?

Similar questions are being raised about the appropriate age for a woman to have a mammography. A thirty-eight-year-old secretary, the first in her family to have breast cancer, had a mastectomy when she was thirty-two and has had a mammography every year since. "The chance of not having the mammography is more of a risk and fear to me than the radiation." Another woman in her late thirties whose mother had had breast cancer and who had three benign tumors removed from her own breasts resolved her fear over the risk of getting cancer from x-rays and the risk of letting a malignancy go undetected by having a mammography every other year.

These women are in a high-risk group, generally defined as women under fifty who have had a breast cancer or whose mother or sisters have had it, women with breast lumps, cysts, or nipple discharge. Only 3 to 5 percent of women under fifty have a risk high enough to justify mammography, according to Bailar. American Cancer Society officials disagree. Adding unusually large breasts to the high-risk category, the ACS reported in the *Reader's Digest* that 80 percent of the women under fifty are in a high-risk group for getting breast cancer.

While the debate about who should and should not receive breast x-rays continues, and the confusion about what to do proliferates, the cruelest blow in the mammography muddle was the discovery, in 1977, that, in a review of 506 breast lesions less than one centimeter in size, which the x-rays discovered, sixty-six of the tiny cancer tumors were really benign tumors, and that for twenty-two additional women, minimal cancers were reclassified and called "unclear" or "borderline" tumors. This information came too late; fifty-three of the women had already had mastectomies. Surgery on such small lesions, difficult to analyze pathologically, was hasty, unnecessary, and tragic. Even this discovery was not disclosed without confusion. Two months after the announcement of the errors, the National Cancer Institute reported that "only" seven women had had needless operations. There were, however, thirty more cases on which the NCI's advisory committee of expert pathologists disagreed.

Three years after the screening program began, women were still getting mixed messages about the efficacy of mammographies. By late 1977, the National Cancer Institute and the American Cancer Society issued very strict guidelines, recommending mammographies for women in the thirty-five to thirty-nine year age group *only* if they previously had had cancer in one breast. Just a few months before, they had recommended mammographies for this age group if the woman had had a cancer or if there was a family history of it. Seemingly overnight, the criteria for mammography changed.

Meanwhile, critics now say that the x-ray doses given in many facilities are so high that the break-even point for lives saved from early detection is the age of fifty-five. Bailar now wonders whether older women already at high risk for breast cancer may also be at high risk for induction of radiogenic cancers. "If so, high-risk women may be the least suitable candidates for mammography." Radiologists, however, claim that new, improved machines emit lower, and therefore safer, radiation doses while providing a sharper image.

One short-term solution to the mammography muddle is to use the machine as little as possible until there is more information about it. But that moment of truth seems farther and farther away, as conflicting statements about the risks and benefits of mammography continue to appear.

Repeating Past Errors

The philosophy behind the "use now, evaluate later" theory of new medical technology is compelling. Shoshanna Abeles benefited from the CAT scanner before its widespread use was proven efficacious by clinical studies, and women over fifty whose cancers are discovered by mammography are given a better chance for a longer life even though valid criteria for screening women for breast cancer have not yet evolved.

Although the wisdom of using a new technology before its safety and efficacy are evaluated is highly questionable, historically this is the route that has been chosen. The safety of x-rays, for example, has been questioned since they were first introduced in 1895 by the German physics professor Wilhelm Konrad Roentgen. One physician working with x-rays lost his body hair where he aimed the machine at himself, but, before long, hair loss became one of the least serious problems associated with radiation exposure. X-ray workers began to suffer skin loss, gangrene, and impaired vision, and were soon considered high risks by life insurance companies.

The first American x-ray worker to die from radiation exposure was Thomas Edison's glass-blowing assistant, Clarence Madison Dally, who frequently placed his hands — most often his right hand — in the x-ray beam while testing the tubes he made. Dally developed a large ulcer on his right wrist that failed to heal, in spite of over 100 skin grafts. Eventually both arms were amputated, and he died of cancer in 1904.

Although dangers were inherent from the very beginning, the concept of x-raying was appealing, and it spread widely, rapidly, and often inappropriately, causing both patients and technicians alike to become victims of unnecessary radiation.

Chest x-rays became a standard procedure by the 1920s, and by 1930 were considered the most exact diagnostic technique for tuberculosis. The mere observation of an abnormal density on a lung x-ray could have profound effects on the course of life. A young husband living in New York City would be forced to spend a year or two away from his wife, young children, and his job, while he was hospitalized in the Adirondacks.

The frequent major upheaval of lives for people diagnosed as having TB continued to occur until the late 1940s, when an attempt was made to validate the efficacy of x-rays. Researchers found that physicians often disagreed among themselves about interpreting the information printed on the x-ray. In one third of the cases, the physician would disagree with a second or third reader. Moreover, in 20 percent of the cases, the physician would not even agree with himself; that is, when shown the same pair of x-ray films on two different occasions, he would give diametrically opposing answers.

In the 1940s and 1950s, as many as four million American children underwent x-ray treatments for therapeutic reasons, because of a widely held belief that x-rays could combat tonsillitis and adenoid troubles. The National Cancer Institute reports that people who were treated with x-rays for these conditions when they were children now, as adults, show an alarming tendency toward thyroid cancer.

The Michael Reese Hospital in Chicago began examining adults who had been treated with x-rays when they were young. The hospital found abnormalities of the thyroid in 300 out of the first 1000 persons they examined, and sixty of the abnormalities were subsequently diagnosed as malignant tumors. A still higher incidence of cancer of the thyroid among this group is likely, since 29 percent of those who had abnormalities detected did not return for further testing.

Thyroid cancer is a relatively rare disease, usually occurring in one person out of 27,000, so the data from Michael Reese — a minimum of sixty thyroid cancers in 1000 persons — are both shocking and alarming. The true incidence of thyroid cancer in those who, as youngsters, were treated for tonsillitis and infected adenoids is not known because not all patients have been found. Nor is it likely that they will be found. Records from twenty and thirty years ago have often been destroyed or are not available. Hospital radiologists from those days have for the most part retired or died, and many patients were treated in the private offices of radiologists, where records were not entered into any continuing system. Complicating the issue, many patients have moved, and most females have changed their names.

In spite of the fact that these dangers are documented in medical literature, the overuse of x-rays persists. Researchers at the Massachusetts Institute of Technology stated recently that nearly one third of all x-rays taken are not even medically justified. Rather, they are ordered because the physicians are worried about potential malpractice threats.

In addition to the radiation dangers inherent in unnecessary x-rays, the health-care costs soar for wasteful purposes. It is estimated that medical and dental x-rays cost Americans nearly $5 billion a year. If 30 percent of these are unnecessary, that means that nearly $2 billion are spent for diagnostic procedures that are of no help to the patient. Moreover, pointed out Priscilla W. Laws, a physics professor and consumer advocate for rational use of x-rays, "since the total annual malpractice settlements are only about one hundred million dollars per year, patients are paying fourteen times more for defensive x-rays than they are getting back in settlements from all types of malpractice suits."

X-rays are not the only diagnostic tool that doctors order liberally and without proof of need. A battery of diagnostic procedures performed as part of an annual checkup may take several hours and cost as much as $500. "This expenditure may be justified," according to Harvard Medical School professor of medicine Richard Spark, "if it can be demonstrated that the periodic health examination provides an effective means of maintaining the public's health." Spark, in a highly controversial article in the *New York Times* magazine, argued that the tests find too little and cost too much.

Consider the statistics from a seven-year experiment with more than 10,000 members of the Kaiser-Permanente prepaid health plan, ranging in age between thirty-five and fifty-four. Half the group was urged to have frequent periodic health exams; the other half was not. If there were benefits from having periodic exams, then people in the first group would be expected to have significantly fewer deaths, less disease, and less disability than those in the second group. But the differences between the two groups in terms of mortality, suffering from chronic disease, even time lost from work due to illness, were negligible and statistically insignificant.

"As unpleasant as it may sound to those who would like to believe otherwise, most diseases can be detected only after symptoms appear," concluded Spark. Moreover, according to Spark, there is no convincing evidence that there is any advantage to treating a disease, with the exception of hypertension, before symptoms arise.

In spite of this indictment, there are valuable life-saving routine diagnostic procedures, such as the Pap smear test for cancer of the cervix, screening for hypertension, and the limited use of mammography. But the full range of diagnostic tests is under clear attack.

*

Diagnoses can be made for the functioning of virtually every part of the human body. But what good does it do to identify a symptom when the meaning of it is so poorly understood that some physicians view it as a serious syndrome that could lead to death, others use it as a life-saving diagnostic tool, and a third group calls it a benign curiosity. The diagnosis of systolic click raises all three possibilities.

Systolic click is an extra motion made by the heart with each beat because of a buckling of a main valve in the heart. The click is detected most often in young women. For years, it was either overlooked by physicians listening with a stethoscope or noted by acutely listening cardiologists as an unimportant oddity. Now that it is easily detected by echocardiographs, the same condition that lay dormant for years as an innocent curiosity is being described — and treated — as a full-fledged disease, and it is being associated with chest pain, fatigue, arrhythmias, infection of heart valves, even sudden death.

Joseph Romeo, an internist and heart consultant to the U.S. State Department, recalled the case of one forty-year-old foreign service officer who was told she could not have an overseas post for which she was slated because of her heart condition, systolic click. "Why not restrict two-pack-a-day smokers from overseas posts?" asked Romeo. "They are in greater danger of getting coronary heart disease than is the woman with systolic click."

"Women with systolic click are now being labeled as sick when they are not," according to Washington internist and cardiology specialist Michael J. Halberstam. He questions whether a finding that occurs in approximately 10 percent of young women could be termed a "condition" and whether these women should be called "patients." "My response to all of the above is no . . . If there were truly a systolic click syndrome, healthy young women would be dropping dead all around us. They aren't.

"Medicalization is one of the risks of modern medicine," Halberstam continued. "Because we can identify something, we call it a disease when it is not. Treating women with systolic click as if they had coronary heart disease would be like treating everyone with freckles as if they had melanoma."

*

The bagful of diagnostic tools provides some, but not all, of the answers. Although lives are saved, they are saved at a large social and human cost. The CAT scanner finds many diseases for which there are no cures. Mammograms show tiny cancers that turn out not to be malignant. Echocardiographs detect conditions that are not even diseases. As new diagnostic procedures are developed, they too are likely to be accepted rapidly by both physician and patient before the safety and efficacy of the devices are known. The quest to see more and more of the inner workings of the human body is another of the medical world's attempts to play God. What is lacking is the infallibility of a deity.

Chapter 8

The Body Shop

DOROTHY'S FRIENDS in *The Wizard of Oz* are prototypes of real people in search of medical treatment. The Scarecrow needs a brain and a replenishment of straw for various parts of his body. The Tin Woodman wants a heart and a supply of oil to make his joints work, much as humans need blood to make their bodies work. And the Cowardly Lion has a heart problem he would like to have corrected. "Whenever there is a danger," he whines, "my heart begins to beat fast." Heartbeats are routinely regulated with pacemakers, but the lion thought an infusion of courage would resolve his problem.

Much like Dorothy's friends, humans can consult with a wizard — in the guise of a doctor — to have their lives recharged by adding, technologically, the part of their body that is missing or not operating correctly. Much of the body's innards — kidneys, heart, liver, lungs — can be transplanted. There are false limbs that move, plastic lenses that can see, eardrums that can hear, even artificial penises that can have erections. Machines simulate the functions of the kidneys and liver by cleansing poisons from the blood, and researchers are working on an artificial pancreas that will dole out insulin.

With the development of a wide range of sophisticated body replacements, health care has moved into an exotic area of life-saving therapies in which resources are scarce. This scarcity is in direct conflict with the long-held view of health care as a right on which unlimited demands can be made.

How to allocate these scarce resources is a perplexing dilemma unanticipated by medical traditions. In taking the Hippocratic Oath, for example, a doctor promises to work for the benefit of the sick in "whatsoever house I enter." By swearing to do this, how can a physician make the choice to use an artificial liver machine for saving one person's life but not to use it for saving everyone? With unlimited demands and limited supplies, a selection process is mandatory. Who shall live when not everyone can?

Triage, developed by French medical officers during World War I, divided men into three groups, and those with the best chances of survival were given the best treatment. Based on this theory, soldiers during World War II who were considered as having been "wounded" in brothels, because they had contracted venereal disease, received the scarce supplies of penicillin rather than the men wounded in the field. The reasoning for this allocation was based on utilitarianism. Those who were treated would be of the most help. Military manpower shortage was a critical issue when the first shipment of penicillin arrived at the North African Theater of Operations, U.S.A., in 1943. In less than one week, the men overcrowding the military hospitals with VD were restored to health and returned to battle lines. In contrast, it was months before some of the battle-wounded were well enough to fight.

Or perhaps the most vulnerable people should be treated first. When scientists learned how to isolate insulin from the pancreas in 1920, decisions had to be made about who would receive the limited supplies. Diabetes specialists argued persuasively that the first priority was children, because the mortality rate from diabetes among youngsters was 100 percent.

Is social worth a valid criterion for selecting patients for life-saving technologies? Should a mother of five young children receive a heart transplant rather than a middle-aged bachelor lawyer, or a teen-aged drug addict? Should a brilliant painter likely to make a future contribution to society have any more rights to health care than a day laborer? Or, in the name of equality, should scarce medical resources be awarded to winners of a lottery?

There is no perfect way to deal out scarce resources. Someone will gain, but someone will lose. The treatment of terminal kidney disease illustrates some of the problems American health-care planners have had in trying to grapple equitably with this issue for nearly two decades. The artificial kidney machine, once a scarce resource, is now available to virtually anyone who needs it. No one is denied; everyone lives. But within this changeover from treating a few to treating everyone, the real issue of how to allocate scarce medical resources has not been resolved — either for the treatment of kidney disease or for that of any other disease which requires expensive exotic life-saving technology. The question "Who shall live when not everyone can?" remains unanswered.

The Dialysis Dream . . . and Dilemma

Nancy Karl is full of life. She takes trips to Las Vegas and Israel, spends afternoons at museums and matinées, and writes and edits articles. Nancy is full of life only because she has been on a dialysis machine since her kidneys stopped functioning normally in 1967.

She was twenty-two, and everything for the future looked bright. She had graduated from Barnard College in June, married a young law student, and was working for *Look* magazine. Within a few months, Nancy's future began to look grim. Her ankles became painfully swollen, but she was reassured by her physician that it was a side effect of the birth control pill. That was far from the truth, because her swollen ankles were a sign of impending kidney failure, which took her by surprise in October and caused her to spend three months in the hospital — half of that time in the intensive care unit.

"This illness hit me out of the blue. I was going along my merry way without any warning. The doctors still don't know what caused the failure. My kidneys simply stopped functioning," said Nancy, calmly and knowingly. "And had there not been a kidney machine, I would have been dead years ago."

Temporary dialysis treatments stabilized her condition by mechanically removing toxic wastes from her body — a job normally done by the kidneys. Nancy's kidneys eventually regained some of their ability to function, but they were too scarred to filter out her body's toxic materials properly. She was well enough, however, to go home from the hospital and try to resume a normal life. That was a difficult task: she was always tired, she found it difficult to work, and her marriage broke up.

Two years later, her energy was virtually depleted. Nancy recalls feeling "not well" most of the time. She also had high blood pressure, which was lowered so much with drugs that when she stood up she often fainted. When she fell in the bathroom, got a black eye and a broken front tooth, Nancy realized that she needed someone to take care of her, and she moved back to her parents' home.

She started a new course of treatment with immunosuppressants in an effort to keep her kidneys functoning even minimally. These are the same drugs that are used after transplants to keep organs from being rejected. And it was this course of treatment which convinced Nancy that if her kidneys totally failed, she would return to dialysis for a lifetime, but she would not have a transplant and subject herself to the immunosuppressants again. While on the drugs, she experienced a living nightmare: she hallucinated, heard voices, and became paranoid.

Nancy was sick — but not sick enough to be selected for lifelong use of a dialysis machine. "In those days — the late sixties, early seventies — the machines were reserved for the very sick. You had to be at death's door, with your hands shaking and your head confused, before you could get long-term dialysis treatment."

Nancy reached that point of high confusion and disorientation in 1972, the year she began coming to the dialysis clinic three times a week, as she will continue to do for the rest of her life. In addition, Nancy takes more than a dozen pills a day, to supplement the vitamins, calcium, and iron that are missing from her very rigid diet. Her fluid intake is limited to one quart daily; her proteins are restricted by one-fourth.

"It is nothing that I would ever choose for myself, but I would sure as hell rather be here three times a week than dead," she said. "I know that I have to come here, but I don't think of myself as being dependent on a machine. It has not taken over my life. When I'm not here, I do what I want — and when. For example, when I went to Israel, I did what most tourists do, except for having my dialysis treatments in Beersheba.

"What I miss the most is having a choice. If you're working and don't want to go in one day, you just call in and say you're sick. But I don't have that choice. I have to come in."

Dialysis is the core of Nancy's life, but she realizes that it will not ultimately save her from her disease. "Dialysis is a stopgap measure, not a cure. I have a terminal illness, but when it will be terminal for me, I don't know. I think of everyone's life as terminal. People I went to school with are dead, and here I am — alive."

Nancy Karl's story exemplifies many of the dreams as well as dilemmas of a life on a dialysis machine. She amasses an annual medical bill of $30,000, lives with the constrictions of drink and diet, and functions within the limitations of a chronic disease. Yet Nancy lives, and can live indefinitely, with a terminal illness from which she would have died years before, without dialysis.

*

Dialysis is a classic halfway technology. It keeps a patient alive but can neither cure nor prevent the disease. It was developed in the early 1940s; the first machine was made, from an old bathtub, spare automobile parts, and sausage casings,

by a Dutch physician, Willem J. Kolff, now associated with
the University of Utah in Salt Lake City. Kolff saw his
mechanical kidney as a short-term measure to help patients
through a crisis of temporary kidney failure. While he
watched a patient die from chronic kidney failure, Kolff
thought, "If only I could remove every day as much urea as
he produces, he could live forever."

The major obstacle in using dialysis on a patient forever was
vascular access. Two lifelines are needed to connect the patient to the machine: one to carry the blood from an artery
out of the body, where it can be purified by the dialysis process; the other to return the cleansed blood to a vein. Each time
patients were dialyzed in the 1940s and fifties, they had to
undergo surgery to have tubes inserted in arteries and veins.
This involved the risks of infection, blood clotting, and hemorrhaging; but they were acceptable risks for acutely ill people
who needed dialysis treatments only until they passed over
their medical crisis. Using dialysis on a long-term basis, however, posed too many problems to make it feasible. Not only
were the risks too great, but there were not enough sites on
arms and legs for continually puncturing patients in order to
connect them with the machine.

By 1960, Dr. Belding Scribner, of the University of Washington Medical School in Seattle, devised methods to assure
safe and easy vascular access by implanting two small plastic
tubes in the forearm. One led to a vein, the other to an artery,
and both could be hooked up to the machine. Between hook-
ups, the tubes were kept closed with a U-shaped shunt, which
lay flush on the skin. The shunt system made possible the
transition from short-term use of the dialysis machine to long-
term use. The shunt was eventually replaced by an even sim-
pler and safer process: a vein and an artery were tied together
to make a passageway called a fistula, which could be repeatedly punctured for connection to the machine.

In November 1962, a feature story in *Life* magazine, by
Shana Alexander, reported the glories of the dialysis machine
as a means of saving the lives of victims of chronic kidney

failure. Millions of Americans also learned through the article — dramatically titled "They Decide Who Lives, Who Dies" — the problems of rationing access to the machines. Not everyone with kidney failure could go on dialysis, because the expensive machine was in very limited supply.

The Seattle God Committee — officially called the Admissions and Policies Committee of the Seattle Artificial Kidney Center at Swedish Hospital — was an attempt to grapple with the issue of allocation of scarce resources. The committee met several times a year to decide which patients would get to use the dialysis machine, which ones would not. Those whom they chose would live; those whom they rejected would die.

The committee was made up of seven people who did their jobs anonymously and without pay. It included a lawyer, minister, banker, housewife, an official of state government, a labor leader, and a surgeon. They were asked not to make medical decisions, since all prospective patients would be prescreened by a board of physicians. And they were given only two guidelines: to reject children and people over forty-five.

The committee was given the responsibility of substantially narrowing the field of candidates. "Where do we begin? The universe? The solar system? The earth?" asked one committee member. Finally they agreed to consider only applicants who were residents of the State of Washington, because the basic research to develop the shunt had been done at state-supported institutions. The people whose taxes paid for the research, reasoned the members, should be its first beneficiaries.

Limiting patients to state residents was an arbitrary but relatively easy decision for the God Committee. The patients they excluded were statistical patients — they were numbers, not personalities. The remaining deliberations — those dealing with identifiable people — were far more difficult. There was a housewife living in the northern part of the state who would have to move with her husband and two children to Seattle to receive treatment, a move the family could not really afford. There was an aircraft worker, with six children, who was eager to work but too sick to stay on the job. And there was a chemist and an accountant — each sick but still working. Which of these patients should be selected? Is a person's social worth or family status, even where a person lives, an important criterion for being a candidate for survival?

"I guess that as long as facilities are not unlimited, somebody has to pick and choose," said a small businessman who was eventually selected for the machine. "What a dreadful decision! Frankly, I'm surprised the doctors were able to round up seven people who were willing to take the job."

The storm of criticism aroused by the God Committee led to its fairly rapid demise, and the problem of patient selection still has not been resolved. "The Seattle group was pilloried — which may have been warranted, because no one knows how to compute social worth," said Richard Rettig, a health-care analyst for the RAND Corporation. "But at least they tried to come to grips with the problem as a social one, not a medical one. Most dialysis centers made decisions by burying them in the medical process."

The arbitrary selection among patients competing for limited treatment facilities was finally deemed "no longer tolerable" by the federal government, and, in 1972, Congress agreed to pay most of the costs of treatment for end-stage renal disease (ESRD) through Medicare funds.

After the government stepped in, dialysis was no longer something for the chosen few. Decisions were deferred, and everyone was put on dialysis. In 1967, there were only 700 dialysis patients. By 1972, when the legislation was enacted, there were 6000 patients being kept alive on dialysis. And by 1977, there were 37,000 adults and children receiving care under the federal end-stage renal disease program — most of them dialysis patients — leaving a nearly $1 billion bill for the government. There seems to be no limit, with projections calling for a program that will care for 96,000 persons by 1990, at an expense to the government of more than $4 billion a year.

Although the program was conceived as a charitable gesture, it has ended up as a profitable venture. It costs only an average of $7000 a year to dialyze at home, in contrast to $24,000 at a dialysis center, but there is little money in home dialysis for doctors who are being dubbed "kidney millionaires" because they receive $200 a month in federal reimbursements for each patient treated at a center. As a result, the number of patients on home dialysis has dropped from 40 percent before the government began its reimbursement program to less than 20 percent, and fewer than 10 percent of new patients are even training for home care. Profit-making dialysis centers, in contrast, are beginning to proliferate, and about 20 percent of all dialysis patients are enrolled in facilities managed by *one* for-profit corporation: National Medical Care and Biomedical Applications.

The ethical issue of the sixties — an inquiry into the morality of how a committee can decide who should get scarce life-saving resources — shifted in the late seventies to an inquiry into health-care costs: Is the government morally responsible to pay for terminal kidney disease with a blank check?

*

"There is an obligation to dialyze anyone who wants it," asserted Dr. Peter Berkman, chief of renal diseases at the Washington Hospital Center. "A woman comes here two times a week to be dialyzed. She has cirrhosis of the liver in addition to her kidney problem, and she frequently hemorrhages and has constant diarrhea. She lives in a nursing home and is unlikely ever to live outside it, even though she is only in her early fifties. But if she wants dialysis, why shouldn't she get it?

"The potential for abuse is too great if we decided to play God for just one minute — making judgments about which patients are worthy of getting dialysis and which ones are not, or which cancer patients are so terminal that they should not get dialysis," Berkman said. "And so we end up dialyzing people who perhaps, in a rehabilitative sense, should not be dialyzed. They won't add anything to society, they won't work, won't raise or take care of a family. But they do have a right to be dialyzed."

Suppose physicians were to make the choice as to who gets dialysis. How would they know they are making the right choice? Consider the case of eighty-year-old Thomas Hawkins, who developed kidney disease late in life. Being weak and ill depressed him severely, and the hospital psychiatrist questioned whether he was too old to adjust to the rigors of dialysis. How old is "too old"? Should a severely depressed, sick old man be put in a position of possibly becoming more depressed on dialysis? While the psychiatrist pondered the dilemma, Mr. Hawkins was put on dialysis, his depression lifted, and he lived for three more years, with an acceptable and satisfying existence. Yet in the days of limited dialysis machines, the Seattle God Committee would have excluded Mr. Hawkins as a dialysis candidate because of his age.

With the advent of federal financing of dialysis, there are few contraindications for its use. People once thought of as poor candidates for dialysis — those who were too old, too young, or too sick — are now considered acceptable. A senile woman, for example, is transported three times a week, at a cost of $75 for each round trip, from her nursing home to the dialysis unit. "Is this kind of life worth living?" questioned psychiatrist Charles Tartaglia, a consultant for dying heart, cancer, and kidney patients at the Georgetown University Hospital. "Worth living for whom? Are we doing harm to a patient? The family? To society? Is life worth living at any price? My own feeling is that it probably is not. But I am one step removed. I am healthy and am not in the position of having to make that decision about myself."

When Lee Foster, assistant travel editor of the *New York Times* and a three-times-a-week dialysis patient, was asked how it felt to spend so much time hooked up to a blood-cleansing machine, he responded, "Great, when you consider the alternative." Foster spent two years on dialysis before he died of complications from a replacement of a hip joint. (Many patients with terminal kidney disease also suffer from orthopedic problems because calcium is restricted in their diet.)

Foster coped well with dialysis, but it depressed Dan Jones, a recent magna cum laude graduate who had majored in psychology. "I would like to do counseling for patients," he said. "I've had renal problems since I was eighteen months old, and certainly have had enough experience observing sick people. But dialysis is my career now. I'm too tired to do anything else. A person needs to do more than just exist on a machine." (The average time per week spent by people on dialysis, including travel to and from a center, is thirty-seven hours.)

There is nothing wrong with Jones's perceptions: dialysis *is* depressing as a way of life. A recent study revealed that dialysis is so depressing that the suicide rate among people on the machine is more than 100 times the normal rate. Of 3500 patients, there were eighteen successful suicide attempts and nineteen cases of voluntary withdrawal from dialysis (and therefore death), a significant increase over the normal suicide rate of ten per one hundred thousand.

Since equity of treatment does not necessarily result in equity of outcome, should the quality of life be a criterion in deciding who should use an expensive medical technology such as dialysis? Only 40 percent of the dialysis patients are rehabilitated to the point where they have a good quality of life, where they can engage in their normal activities, as does Nancy Karl. Twenty-eight percent will continue to feel chronically ill, as does Dan Jones; and the rest — 32 percent — will die within three years after treatments begin.

The Alternative of Transplants

All this time, money, physical and psychological pain — and less than 50 percent of the dialysis patients live long enough to enjoy life. Is this the best that modern medicine can offer for a projected bill of $4 billion a year?

Until recently, there was a fairly limited set of options open to a person when a particular bodily function ceased to operate properly. The organ could spontaneously revive itself; the malfunctioning could be treated with drugs (diuretics, for example, can control some kidney disease) or with mechanical appliances, such as dialysis machines. Add transplants to this growing list of options — and the growing list of ethical concerns in medicine.

*

Soon after she began college, Gay Polyzois learned she had a kidney disease. She never thought of it as anything serious, and for six years it was under control with diuretic drugs. During that time she completed college, received a graduate degree in French studies, and traveled to Europe — including a trip back to her family's home in Greece. She eventually started to lose her energy, had no appetite, even had difficulty walking. And by 1974, all her normal activities stopped when her kidneys ceased functioning.

Gay began a new way of life — hooking herself up to a dialysis machine three times a week. Though it saved her life at the time, dialysis was not a long-term solution for Gay. She developed congestive heart failure, contracted hepatitis, hallucinated, had dangerously high blood pressure, and temporarily lost her eyesight. Dialysis was barely keeping her alive, but it did its job well enough until she found a suitable donor for a kidney transplant.

Fortunately for Gay, her mother was both a willing and well-matched donor. Plans were made for Mrs. Polyzois to give her daughter a kidney, but the night before the scheduled transplantation, pathologists found blood in a sample of Mrs. Polyzois's urine and traced it to a kidney stone. Since good health and perfectly functioning kidneys are requisites for a donor, Gay's mother was no longer an acceptable candidate.

But Gay's younger sister, Connie, was also a willing and well-matched donor. "I was so worried about my sister," said Gay. "What if kidney disease runs in the family? If she gives me a kidney and her remaining one fails, poor thing would end up on a machine like me. I was so tired and so depressed. I was really ready to die. I felt that my life was shattered — finished. Why should she jeopardize her life for me?"

But Connie gave her kidney to Gay, and now, two years

later, both sisters are doing well. Gay is alive, full of energy, grateful for the "chance Connie took to see me well again," and for the advances in medicine that permitted her to outlive her defective kidneys.

The price Gay pays is doses of cortisone and immunosuppressants, for the rest of her life, to counteract her body's natural impulse to reject foreign tissues. There are some obvious physical signs of superficial importance — thinning hair, puffy cheeks, and acne. The nonvisible signs of the drugs she takes are more life-threatening: they lower her white blood cell count, so she is susceptible to many diseases. So far, Gay has not become seriously ill, but there is a chance that the drugs will lower her resistance to some common virus and that she will succumb to it.

"Everything done for me is experimental," Gay acknowledged. "That's how progress is made in the medical field. How do they know that the drug I've been taking won't do something bad later on? I'm a prime target for cancer because of the drugs, but I don't worry about that. What's important now is keeping alive."

Gay's main worry is that the kidney will be rejected. Although 80 to 90 percent of the kidneys implanted from related donors are functioning well after two years, in contrast to a 50 percent success rate for transplants from nonrelated donors, a rejection could occur at any time. Unlike a heart transplant, rejection of a kidney does not mean death. But it does mean that the patient must return to dialysis.

"I couldn't go back to the machine," said Gay. "I can't see staying on it again, getting congestive heart failure or going blind. I had too many unpleasant experiences on it to go back to the machine." But Gay holds on to a wedge to keep the door of life open: "I might go back on it for a short time only — to wait for a cadaver transplant."

*

While most patients prefer life as a transplantee to the experiences of living on chronic dialysis, not everyone is as lucky as Gay Polyzois. Sixteen-year-old Steve Leahy has been on dialysis for three years and is literally dying to get off it. He had one transplant, which his body rejected, and offers of dozens of other kidneys, none of which matched his body's antigens.

"Steve is a tough kid," said his mother, Jean Leahy, "and when he lost his donor kidney, he was very depressed. For the first time, he really showed strong emotions about his disease [a hereditary form of nephritis]. He talks coolly about death and knows he will die young. But he doesn't like to be tied down. It's hard for him to be back on dialysis — a real tying-down experience. And it's hard to be cool when you're on dialysis."

Meanwhile, Steve waits for another suitable donor.

Just before Christmas, Jean Leahy received a phone call from the hospital: a kidney was available from someone who had died and had the same blood type and some of the antigens that both Steve and his brother Tom have. Tom suffers from the same fatal kidney disease, but he is not as sick as Steve. In fact, Steve was so sick the day the kidney arrived that he could not have withstood the trauma of the major surgery involved in a kidney transplant. Tom received the kidney instead.

A God Committee does not decide from on high as to who gets a kidney, the way the Seattle group labored over who got dialysis. Strict medical criteria are used: who matches the kidney best, who is sickest, who is least likely to survive on dialysis. If Steve Leahy was given a poor match just because the surgeon felt sorry for him and wanted to see him get a kidney, it would probably be rejected — and therefore wasted.

There are at least 10,000 sufferers of kidney disease in the U.S. waiting for a transplant, yet only 4000 will get one. Three quarters of those receiving a transplant do not have relatives willing or able to donate a kidney, as did Gay Polyzois, so they must wait for one from a dying accident victim. The largest single source of kidneys is healthy people who have had the bad luck to die in an accident — a highway crackup, a homicide, an electrocution. There are more than 100,000 potential suitable cadaver donors each year from accidents such as these, yet organs from only 3 percent of them are transplanted.

The Uniform Anatomical Gift Act, signed by most states in 1970, makes it legally possible for a person to will a body to medicine, the way one wills property to heirs. But the Uniform Donor Card — the piece of paper that permits the kidneys to be legally removed at the time of death — is a well-kept secret. More than ten million have been distributed, but few card-carrying donors actually end up giving their organs for transplants. States are beginning to follow the lead of Illinois, Tennessee, and Maryland in handing out donor cards with a driver's license so that motorists can approve signing over their organs in case of accidental death.

There are several reasons why donor cards do not result in more kidney donations. Medical personnel don't always look for the cards; physicians often require approval of next of kin to remove an organ even if a person carries a card; and people are reluctant to desecrate a body and give away a dead relative's organs. "It is not pleasant for us to approach families in grief — but we must do it," said Dr. Charles Currier, a Washington transplant surgeon. "Some people wait for more than two years for a kidney. Only by approaching families can we help reduce the number of patients waiting."

Another factor inhibiting the donation of kidneys is the murky issue of defining death. Without a universally accepted definition of death, many physicians and most hospital administrators are fearful of lawsuits and cautious about removing kidneys from the brain-dead, even with the consent from close family members.

The issue of the scarcity of available kidneys was dramatically highlighted in March 1977, when the kidney of a sixteen-year-old Russian youth killed in an automobile accident in Moscow was transplanted forty-eight hours later into a Brooklyn construction worker in an operation in New York City. In Russia, physicians universally define death as the end of brain activity (less than one fourth of the states have agreed to this definition). Also, Russian physicians do not have to ask next of kin for permission to remove an organ, and malpractice suits are virtually unknown. While the Soviet pattern is not the American way, wider endorsement of the brain-death criterion by state legislatures could be helpful in correlating the ethics of the need for usable organs with the rights of the dying patient.

*

From expensive dialysis machines to card-carrying precadavers, the current methods for controlling kidney disease do little to cure it. The technology for treating kidney disease attacks the public's imagination and pocketbook, but prevention could save more people's lives.

"A lousy thirty-five-cent urine test could help keep a lot of children from getting end-stage renal disease," said Dr. Frederick Green, of the Children's Hospital in Washington. "Acute chronic urinary tract problems have their genesis in early childhood. Some of them could be prevented by health education, but preventive detection could do wonders. A urine analysis done regularly in childhood could significantly cut down on terminal kidney disease later in life. The problem with American medicine is that we are so enamored with technology and with a disease orientation that we pay too little attention to preventive medicine."

Prevention deals with statistical lives — those who might get the disease — not identifiable lives — those who will die without dialysis treatments. The priorities are clear. In the late 1970s, federal spending on treatment was nearing $1 billion, but research into better understanding of kidney disease, so that it could be prevented, received less than $50 million.

Getting to the Heart of the Matter

The thirty million American victims of heart disease have neither the assurances of a medical technology like dialysis to extend their lives nor the luxury of a federally guaranteed blank check to buy their way out of sickness. Yet more than 70,000 people a year with heart pain are spending $1 billion for major surgery that may not even be of help. Coronary artery bypass surgery holds a promise, but is not a foolproof method, for treating coronary arteries that are clogged, a condition that can cause great pain as well as death. The surgery creates a bypass for the parts of the coronary arteries that are severely or totally obstructed. One end of a vein, taken from the leg, is sewn to the aorta; the other end is attached to the coronary arteries.

The benefits of bypass surgery have not been completely demonstrated and validated, and claims that the operation prevents death remain largely unproven. Yet patients weighed down by the fear of death from the nation's leading killer — and spurred on by testimonials from those who have had the surgery — are seeking the operation.

Fear is a major factor in a person's having bypass surgery. Cardiologist Richard S. Ross, dean of the Johns Hopkins University Medical School, told the Senate Human Resources Subcommittee on Health and Scientific Research that 25 percent of the operations are done on the mistaken assumption that patients will be less likely to have a heart attack or die suddenly. Although many patients claim that bypass relieves chest pain, it reappears in 40 percent of the cases, and "there is no evidence that the operation prevents sudden death or makes patients with coronary artery disease live longer," Ross testified.

The costs of the bypass operation are high in terms of money, lives, and medical know-how. The operation costs $12,500 and carries with it a 1 to 3 percent risk of death and a 4 percent chance of inducing a heart attack. Even before surgery, the patient is at risk, because two in every 1000 die as a result of arteriography, a diagnostic procedure in which dye is injected into the coronary blood vessels to determine which arteries are blocked and to what extent.

In an attempt to evaluate the benefits and risks of coronary artery bypass, and to suggest when it is appropriately needed,

Veterans' Administration researchers studied 600 patients with angina heart pain. After treating half with drugs and half with surgery, the VA team found no statistical difference in the overall health of the men in either patient group. Eighty-eight percent of the men who had had the bypass operation were alive three years later. For the same time period, 87 percent of the men treated with drugs survived. In one type of heart problem, however, there was an increased survival rate because of the bypass surgery: 92 percent of the men with left main artery disease were still living eighteen months after the operation; only 70 percent of the men who had the same condition but were treated solely with drugs were still alive. In this condition, the main coronary artery serving the lower left chamber of the heart — the part of the heart that gives blood its final push into the body's circulation system — gets clogged.

"In medicine, there is a tendency to jump onto new bandwagons," said Dr. Joseph Romeo, "and when bypass was first introduced in nineteen sixty-seven, many physicians became very enthusiastic. Everyone needed it. No one was expendable. It has taken ten years to sort out this new therapy. Sanity is returning to the way heart doctors are practicing. We are now selecting good surgical candidates for bypass — like those with left main artery disease. Before, we didn't know who were good surgical candidates."

*

Surgery and mechanical interventions such as pacemakers, which electrically regulate the heartbeat, can help alleviate some of the complications of coronary heart disease. But for some patients, the only alternative to death is a live heart transplant.

The hope of transplants was held out to men and women with heart problems when Louis Washansky, a South African grocer, made medical history in 1967 by having the first human heart transplant. Washansky lived only eighteen days, but Emmanuel Vitria, a Frenchman who received a heart in 1968, was still alive a decade later. Statistically, heart transplants are not successful enough to provide a meaningful option for heart disease. Only 20 percent of the patients survive more than one year.

The accounting for heart transplants is askew: costs are high (as much as $50,000), and survivorship is low. Individuals are free to choose whatever therapy they want, but should the federal government be morally obligated to finance it? Should we even permit the "most skilled surgeons to devote their resources to techniques that have a very low degree of success?" asked Robert Veatch, an ethicist at the Hastings Center in Hastings-on-Hudson, New York. "There may well be more useful things that can be done with their skills."

Yet another choice for sufferers of coronary heart disease will soon be available: the totally implantable artificial heart. Materials for the artificial heart are still being perfected, since most of the synthetics are incompatible with blood and could cause fatal clotting. The power source to keep the heart operating must also be refined. Options include pellets of plutonium, batteries that can be recharged through the skin, and biological fuel cells, which operate with glucose in the blood and would be refueled every time a person ate.

An atomic scientist and consultant to the National Heart and Lung Institute (NHLI), which developed the artificial heart, worries about the radiation hazards to the public from a plutonium-238–powered heart pump. He fantasizes about going on a six-hour flight and sitting between two people with nuclear-powered hearts. Though the radiation risks to the public are not known, the risk of nearly two ounces of plutonium, even though well shielded in the body, would unquestionably be great to the individual with an implanted artificial heart. The chances of that person's developing cancer are high, and sterilization would be likely to occur not only in the recipient but also in his or her spouse.

An artificial heart has kept blood pumping and circulating in a calf for as long as half a year, and a left heart assist — a pump that lowers ventricular pressure and assumes a major portion of the work of the left heart — has already been tested on humans. Few have survived longer than a week.

Medical technologists are predicting success with totally implantable artificial hearts by the turn of the century, and inquiries into the legal, ethical, psychological, and economic implications have already begun. The question of allocation — who will receive the artificial heart — is initially being resolved the way the dialysis issue was: everyone will get it. Because the device was developed with public money — it has been financed through the NHLI since 1965 — the patient's value to society and the ability to pay should have no place as selection or exclusion criteria, concluded a special ethics committee convened by the American Medical Association. And a report of the President's Biomedical Research Panel agrees that "as with the kidney, it seems very likely that we will insist that no individual should die for want of an artificial heart once it becomes available. Criteria instead would be based solely on medical need."

Costs for the artificial heart will be predictably high: the NHLI estimates that each heart will cost $25,000 and that there would be some 50,000 hearts implanted each year, at an aggregate cost of some $1 billion annually. When does medical care become so costly that federal financing becomes an imperative? When does a procedure become so expensive that the federal government can no longer afford to finance it?

The government is already spending $1 billion a year for treating kidney disease, a figure that will soar to $4 billion by 1990. And there is the potential for another billion dollars a year for an implanted artificial heart. Is there no end to health-care expenditures? The Institute of Medicine, in a report entitled "Disease by Disease Toward National Health Insurance," finds these vast expenditures on palliative approaches to health care to be "curious," and challenges the ethics of government funding of health care. Money funneled into the development of these technologies, argues the institute, would not be available for important areas of research. Yet only through research can we get at the cause of these diseases and develop medical interventions that are far less expensive and that avert long-term disability. How many billions of dollars would the nation still be spending on iron lungs if the research for the prevention of polio had not been done?

The kidney disease decision is the first in a long line of decisions that will be made about the expenses and responsibilities of health care. "The single most important thing that society must learn from this," said Dr. James C. Hunt, president of the National Kidney Foundation, "is to take a stand on extraordinary care, because there just aren't enough resources to provide all the care everybody needs. And they can't leave the whole issue up to doctors. Society has to take a role."

III

DEATH

Chapter 9

Postponing Death

DEATH TAKES PLACE TODAY in an age of technology in which few limits are placed on efforts to extend life. From the treatment of half-formed babies with no ability to breathe independently to that of eighty-five-year-old senile terminal cancer patients, there is a seemingly endless list of medical wonders that can be used to postpone death.

But how much can death really be postponed? What if nobody died of cancer, the disease that 80 percent of Americans fear more than any other? What if the federal government's heralded War on Cancer, in which nearly $1 billion is spent annually to detect causes and cures of the disease, is won?

Then the 400,000 people dying each year of cancer would die of something else. Actuaries report that if cancer were eliminated as a cause of death, the average life expectancy would be increased by a mere 2.5 years for those under thirty-five years of age. And for those sixty-five years old, the expectation of life would be increased by only 1.4 years.

"If you believe that the worst thing is to die of cancer," said surgeon Glenn Geelhoed at the George Washington University Medical Center in Washington, D.C., "then we can try to change that for you with surgery, chemotherapy, radiation, and immunotherapy. But then you will have to die of something else."

And if there is no disease to confound one's efforts to live on, each person will die, after all, of old age. "Old ones come to be dead," wrote Gertrude Stein in *The Making of Ameri-*

cans. "Any one coming to be an old enough one comes to be a dead one." Pneumonia used to be the friend of the old ones, but now it no longer steals them away, as diseases are kept at bay with medical technologies that help maintain virtually every part of their bodies. More sophisticated medical interventions will be developed to avert the aging process and to postpone death further — perhaps the reprogramming of genes through advances in genetic engineering, insertion of chemicals to promote longer-living cells, or replacement of poorly functioning hearts with implanted artificial ones.

Death is now a changing concept because of medical technological interventions. The way of dying, the time of dying, even the signs of dying, have been altered. The classic indications that death has taken place — no breath on a mirror, no heartbeat or pulse — are no longer valid in some circumstances, since a respirator can keep a moribund person breathing indefinitely, and a heart-lung machine can provide respiratory and circulatory functions at least temporarily. Robert Veatch foresees the development of an efficient, compact heart-lung machine capable of being carried on the back or even in a pocket of a person whose heart and lungs are permanently nonfunctioning. "Some might consider such a technological man an affront to human dignity," Veatch said. "Some might argue that such a device should never be connected to a human; but even they would, in all likelihood. agree that such people are alive."

The technical ability to keep people alive clouds the ethical issue of whether they *should* be kept alive. When physicians at the time of Hippocrates wrestled with the problem of not knowing how far they should go in trying to heal a very sick body, they relied on the classic Greek principle of restraint, and they refused to treat "those who are overmastered by their diseases, realizing that in such cases medicine is powerless."

Physicians, moralists, theologians, and others concerned with the sanctity of life and the rights of the dying are wrestling with a modern version of the same problem when they debate whether to resuscitate people who are "overmastered by their diseases." Pope Pius XII grappled with the problem of the morality of resuscitation when he said, in a public statement in 1957, that man has a duty to preserve life and health, but is obliged to use only ordinary means to achieve this end — those which do not impose ponderous hardships on oneself or on others.

Ordinary means, in this context, signify those in keeping with the circumstances of the person, place, time, and culture. Using antibiotics for pneumonia is an ordinary means of medical practice, and failure to give these drugs could be construed as medical negligence — and tantamount to killing — if the patient died but could have been restored to good health with the drugs. But withholding antibiotics from a patient who develops pneumonia *in addition* to an illness that can no longer be controlled — say, a terminal liver cancer, which has spread to other parts of the body — is not considered killing, but rather is thought of as letting a person die.

The pope stated that physicians are not obligated to use extraordinary means — specifically, modern respiratory technology — in cases "considered to be completely hopeless" by the physician and when the treatment would go against the wishes of the family. The scenario becomes more difficult if a person is already on the respirator when this irreversible, hopeless state is declared, and the act of shutting off the life-sustaining equipment causes the patient's heart to stop beating. Nevertheless, the act of pulling the plug, according to the pope, should be considered neither a direct cause of death nor a direct assault on the life of the patient.

The decision as to when death takes place — in contrast to whether it should take place — was appropriately left to the medical profession. And in 1968 the Harvard Medical School Ad Hoc Committee to Examine the Definition of Brain Death tried to resolved the problem by establishing criteria for declaring a person brain-dead even though other bodily functions are still operating, albeit with help from extraordinary measures. The criteria have been accepted by several states and have been the basis of numerous court decisions.

The Harvard criteria rely on four facts that must be confirmed — and reconfirmed twenty-four hours later: (1) a total unresponsiveness in the patient, even to the most intensely painful stimuli; (2) no movements or independent breathing; (3) no reflexes, in combination with fixed and dilated pupils; and (4) the most controversial element in the criteria — a flat reading on the electroencephalogram (EEG), indicating the absence of brain activity.

The lack of brain waves as one of the proofs of brain death has been verified by more than 3500 flat EEG readings taken from patients who never again regained consciousness. However, the test is not foolproof. An Ontario neurologist made a brain-wave analysis of a blob of lime Jell-O and obtained readings that could be mistaken as evidence of life. The EEG experiment was made in the intensive care unit, and the squiggly line it produced reflected stray electrical signals given off by nearby respirators, intravenous feeders, and human activity.

Neurologists are searching for other criteria to ascertain whether or not a person is brain-dead. A likely alternative is the criterion developed by a Scandinavian group of physicians, which declares a person brain-dead after twenty-five minutes, based on the absence of blood flow in the brain.

In order to determine this lack of blood flow, a cerebral angiography must be performed, a procedure that involves injecting an opaque dye into the patient and then photographing the brain's blood vessels. If the person is alive, dye would flow through the body and into the brain vessels. If blood vessels are not visible on the angiogram, then it is proof that blood circulation has not taken place since the time the dye was injected, and that the patient is brain-dead. Performing the invasive diagnostic test of cerebral angiography adds one more burdensome technological insult to those who are dying — perhaps even dead.

Gleaning information from the brain-death criteria is not the same as making a decision about how to treat a patient and when to stop using life-prolonging measures. When an EEG was given to Karen Ann Quinlan, a twenty-one-year-old New

Jersey woman who went into a coma after mixing alcohol and drugs on the night of April 15, 1975, physicians found that she did not meet the criteria for death. Her brain had minimal capacities to maintain the vegetative aspects such as the regulation of blood pressure and swallowing. But it had lost its cognitive capabilities, those which make it possible for a person to talk, think, see, and feel.

She was alive, but the mechanical respirator was unplugged a year later, after the New Jersey Supreme Court ruled that Karen's parents could assert a right to privacy for her and request cessation of the life-sustaining technology. The court, in making its decision,wrote that "the law, equity, and justice must not themselves quail and be helpless in the face of modern technological marvels presenting questions hitherto unthought of."

Karen was removed from the respirator in March 1976 but was not left to die in a natural state. At the request of her parents, she was given high-nutrient feedings and antibiotics for her recurrent infections. She was also turned periodically, to prevent the formation of bed sores, and was carefully monitored by physicians and nurses in a nursing home, where she lay with few signs of passing from her nether world between life and death. As this book is being written, Karen Quinlan has remained in that state for more than two years. Death, when it comes, will be a technological event, not a natural one.

*

While the age of medical technology continues to flourish, there are more and more plugs to turn off and techniques to employ before all hope is given up. A man with liver problems follows simple medical treatments for years — for example, he takes bile salts to help absorb food and to clear up a mild jaundice condition — and ends his days with terminal liver failure, hooked up to a dialysislike liver perfusion machine. A woman with circulatory deficiencies takes digitalis to increase her cardiac output, which in turn improves the blood flow throughout her body. After fifteen years of drug therapy, her condition has deteriorated to the point where a heart-lung machine is the only way to keep her blood pumping. A totally implanted artificial heart, when it is perfected, could help prolong her life even further, but eventually she will die, and morticians will have to invade her body to remove the source of power that keeps her heart beating.

There are technological interventions to forestall the time of death for virtually every life-threatening condition. Even the dead are willing to wait for technological advances. A California physician who was dying of lung cancer requested that his body be put in cold storage — and thawed out when a cure for his disease is found.

Dying isn't easy when technology intervenes.

A Case of Not Giving Up

Stanley Wilks was forty-four years old when he died in the summer of 1977 — after nine months of being drastically ill, after nine months of radical efforts to save his life, and after nine months of intensive care, which cost nearly a quarter of a million dollars.

The cause of Mr. Wilks's illness eluded the medical staff at the George Washington University Medical Center, but they persisted in their efforts to save him because of their great faith in medical technology. "He did not have a malignant disease, and if we could have only found out what was wrong, he could have returned to the kind of life he had led before he got sick," commented Dr. Geelhoed, one of the physicians who treated him.

Wilks, a mathematician with the army, father of four children, and a man usually in good health, complained about pains of indigestion in the fall of 1976. Being a cautious man, he discussed this pain with his doctor and had an electrocardiogram, to make sure his heart was working properly — which it was. But the day before Hallowe'en, he had another series of bad chest pains and collapsed on the floor. His wife, Jocelyn, assumed he was having a heart attack.

But Stanley did not have anything that simple to detect: he was diagnosed as having an inflammation of the pancreas, though doctors never found the cause of this flare-up.

What his doctors did discover early on was that Stanley Wilks was very, very sick. One lung was infected, and he had a pseudocyst on his pancreas, which meant that the pancreas was essentially eating itself up. The cyst blocked the normal flow of digestive enzymes from the pancreas, so the enzymes began digesting the pancreas itself and would soon spread out to "eat" nearby organs. The temporary solution was the insertion of several tubes to drain the excess juices from his pancreas. Surgery to remove the pancreas was too risky: it carries a 10 percent chance of death in otherwise healthy individuals, and surgeons reasoned that the chance of mortality would be much greater for someone in as weak a condition as Wilks. A pancreatectomy posed additional problems. His surgeon, Dr. Geelhoed, explained, "Assuming his survival, which is why we would have wanted to operate, Wilks would have become a diabetic since insulin is produced in the pancreas. He also would have had trouble digesting foods without a pancreas."

Draining the cyst did not solve the problem, and Wilks continued to be very sick, with temperatures running more than 108° F. Placing him between ice blankets cooled his body, but could not control the cause of the recurring fevers. By Christmas he was losing so much weight and was so weak that it was hard for him to sit up. "Previously there was a limit to the amount of torture we put someone through," said Geelhoed. "If a patient lost fifteen percent of his total body weight, he would die. Now we can prevent patients from reaching that state by giving them a few bottles of 'food' a day — a special liquid diet of amino acids and sugar." Wilks, a six-footer, consumed more than 500 bottles of special hyperalimentation nutrition, and his weight fell only thirteen pounds — from 180 to 167.

What was wrong with Stanley Wilks still eluded his physicians, but they didn't stop seeking. On the theory that there was a pocket of infection in his body, hiding somewhere between his lungs and intestines, surgeons opened him up for investigation. They found a distended gallbladder, some gallstones, but no infection.

Before they could agree where next to search for the cause of his illness, Wilks's body went into high gear. Temperatures of 108°, forty breaths per minute (healthy people usually take fifteen breaths per minute), and a high state of anxiety. In an effort to slow down his body so that it could have a chance to fight off the pancreatitis and the other unknown problems that were sure to kill him, doctors put him in a state of suspended animation for seventy-two days by injecting him with curare. This substance, used by some South American tribes on their blowgun darts to paralyze or kill enemies, can serve as a relaxant. Wilks was relaxed, intentionally, to the point where he was paralyzed and barely conscious. He was unable to move a single muscle or breath without the aid of a respirator. But he was still able to get sicker: he hemorrhaged, went into shock, got infections, and developed toxic reactions to medicines.

"It was a blessing that he didn't know what was going on," recalled Jocelyn. "There were so many IVs and drains coming out that his bedside looked as if it were surrounded by spaghetti."

She shuddered, thinking about those days, but added that she had agreed to permit all of the procedures performed on her husband. "How could he have lived without them?" she asked incredulously. "The hospital staff told me that his major vital organs were compatible with life and were working well — if they could only get rid of the pancreatitis. If he were comatose and had lousy brain waves, major organ failure, and no hope — that would be one thing. But everyone had hope and was convinced that he could get better."

And Glenn Geelhoed remained optimistic. "Clinically speaking, there was no evidence of irreversibility of his condition, even though it might have taken him years to recuperate and regain muscle contraction and coordination. Doctors are usually the last to admit defeat, but even if we wanted to, we couldn't keep a person alive indefinitely. If a person has many problems going, some strengths are needed. And Stanley Wilks had those strengths."

After the curare treatments were stopped, Wilks remained paralyzed for several weeks longer. He was fed by a tube running directly into his gastrointestinal tract, a ploy to give him more calories, which in turn might help him heal faster. And he was given large doses of steroids to treat internal swelling of his body's organs.

Stanley Wilks stopped hemorrhaging, began to cool off, and one day in early April he croaked out from behind his tracheotomy tube, which connected him to the respirator, "I want a chair."

"From nothing, he came awake and wanted to sit in a chair," remembered Jocelyn. "No one could believe that a person could be so ill and still living. And there he was, a few weeks later, sitting up in a chair — reading, laughing, and joking."

The George Washington physicians were considering sending him home in late April, but he had a low-grade fever that he could not shake, and again they were not able to pinpoint its source. "He tried so hard to get well. He wanted to go home so badly," Jocelyn Wilks said. But he never got well. Again he started getting one medical problem after another. He developed blood clots in his legs and was treated with blood-thinner medication; he developed infections in his digestive system and had to go back to liquid feedings. For each problem, the hospital staff could find only a temporary solution.

Late in July he developed high fevers again, and an infection was detected in his blood that physicians could not get rid of, no matter what antibiotics were used. He had a CAT scan of his body, and something suspicious appeared on his lung. But before they could investigate what it was, Stanley Wilks was on a spiral — fevers, shock, back on the respirator. But this time, the spiral was getting out of control. All the systems that had worked before began to fail. There was too much acid accumulating in his blood, and he needed a lot of fluids to combat it. But the fluids he was given went straight to his lungs. Diuretics, which normally leach out excess liquid, did not work because his kidneys were not functioning. And putting him on a dialysis machine would not help because his blood pressure was too low to get his blood moving around the dialysis coils.

"Previously, Stanley had different things fail sequentially. We could treat the one thing at a time. But now so many things were going wrong. We couldn't borrow time against his own body any longer," said Dr. Geelhoed, who admitted that he probably would not have treated Wilks so aggressively if, when he came in nine months earlier, he had been as sick as he was in his final days, with so many parts of his body not working.

Two days later, Stanley Wilks finally succumbed, after nine months of lingering death. Ironically, the inflammation of the pancreas, the initial cause of all his problems, had healed. He died of an abscess on his lung.

"Stanley never gave up hope. His optimism kept him going for so long," said his wife, "but it just wasn't enough to sustain him this last time."

"Yet," added Geelhoed, "he almost made it. It's like making a hundred-yard dash and getting tripped at the ninety-third yard."

Now he is dead: 170 days and $248,486 worth of health care paid for by a $500-a-year prepaid health-maintenance organization policy. The extraordinary cost of Wilks's care will be shared in part by members of his group insurance plan, who will add minimally to a scheduled increase in premiums.

How much health care is one person worth? How much effort should be expended to avoid dying? In Stanley Wilks's case, no one was willing to stop the effort. There was never a time in the nine-month siege — until the last two days — when his case looked hopeless. Even a few weeks before he died, he was out on the hospital balcony with his family, watching the Fourth of July fireworks blasting over the Washington Monument. Was there anything else to do with a man like this except treat him?

"Was Wilks worth our care?" Geelhoed asked. "Was he worth displacing health-care delivery at the grassroots level? Probably not, but those are political decisions, and I do not have the capacity to deliver health to needy people in rural West Virginia. I have a concern for the total health economy, but I was responsible not for the good of the state but for one man. This [all the care] is what Stanley wanted. He never said it wasn't worth the effort. And remember that Stanley Wilks always had a life with potential beyond his stay at the hospital — if only he could have gotten out of it alive."

*

For every patient like Stanley Wilks — a very sick person with the potential to get better with medical interventions — there are those whose deaths are interrupted, sometimes put off indefinitely into a Quinlan-type of nether world, by the same interventions.

The case of Rodney Waldman illustrates the problem. Rodney, a thirty-year-old computer analyst and father of two preschool children, was hanging Christmas-tree lights when he fell off the ladder. He had massive internal bleeding, including bleeding into his brain. For Stanley Wilks, some form of treatment worked — until the very end — but Rodney suffered one medical setback after another without relief. His brain began to swell from hydrocephalus, and the surgeon inserted a shunt to drain the excess fluid. But the shunt caused an infection. A second one was put in, but that one offered little relief because it became clotted. When he had difficulty breathing, Rodney was put on a respirator, but that too did not offer full relief, because he needed to have constant suction of his respiratory passages in order to be comfortable.

"No one was optimistic about him the way we were about Stanley Wilks," said Mary Brady, a nurse in the George

Washington Hospital intensive care unit. "We knew we were not saving anyone viable, and we felt we were burdening his wife.

"The biggest decision concerning his treatment was when there was a big fire in town and eleven seriously burned men came in," Brady related. "We had to triage — put patients who were stable enough out of the ICU to allow the sickest to come in. Rodney Waldman was one of the more stable patients, and a rational decision was made to send him out of the ICU."

The staff had always worried about what would happen to Rodney when he left the more sterile environment of the ICU and the constant care he received there. Would he die of infection? Would he be able to breathe without the constant suction the nurses performed?

Brady had reason to be concerned about Rodney's future. He was weaned off the respirator, but he never really woke up. He is now in a convalescent home and could remain there indefinitely, without improvement. "We do not feel self-satisfaction when we save someone who has such poor brain function as this," commented Brady.

There are thousands of cases like Rodney Waldman's where vigorous efforts to save the patients' lives have brought only remorse and disastrous consequences. One pediatrician recalled the time he "brought a baby back after forty-five minutes, and now it's in an institution for the mentally retarded. I feel deep regrets about this every night. The family has been wrecked by the child."

A neurosurgeon talked about the case of a twenty-eight-year-old policeman who had a fight with his wife, left the house in a rage, and had a near-fatal automobile accident. "The cop was in a coma for three months, but we tended to him diligently and helped him come out of it," the physician remembered. "Now his brain is funny. He walks and talks, but is dull — as if he'd had a lobotomy. He doesn't work and rarely leaves the house. He went back to his family — his twenty-three-year-old wife and baby. Did we do them an injustice by 'saving' him? We are playing with a blind deck of cards and don't know the outcome."

"Patients can be overtreated, and that may be worse than not treating at all," observed Ned Cassem, a Harvard psychiatrist and a Jesuit priest. Using a respirator, for example, will not make a contribution to the primary care of a patient with irreversible liver cancer, nor will full nutrition by IV do anything for the tumor of a person in the throes of death.

One reason for overtreating — a sign of reluctance to give up on a dying patient — is a basic fear of death. California psychologist Herman Feifel interviewed hundreds of people and found that physicians are significantly more afraid of death than either the physically sick or a group of healthy, normal forty-year-olds. Physicians chose their careers for many reasons: to help others, relieve suffering, and study scientific features of illness. For many practitioners there is another reason for becoming a physician: to triumph over disease — and death.

But physicians are beginning to place limits on how much they can do and are questioning whether, in their efforts to restore the patient's health, that health will be sufficiently restored to justify the effort, or will create such a grave inconvenience that the effort could be called "extraordinary means."

"Physicians cannot abdicate their role," affirmed cancer specialist Joseph MacDonald. "They have to know what is kind and what is unkind, and when it is time to stop. We could treat a patient until he's a sixty-pound wreck and justify it medically — but not morally."

Cancer Drugs: A Controversial Way to Extend Life

For many physicians, the big ethics issue in medicine is not whether to pull the plug, but whether to give chemotherapy for cancer. There are more than fifty anticancer drugs on the market today and twice that many being tested on some

30,000 dying men, women, and children. The success of these drugs in curtailing the spread of cancer cannot be denied. But the widespread use of them in clinically unproven situations remains questionable.

The popular appeal of the use of chemotherapies is due to their remarkable success with certain cancers. In the 1940s, the average survival rate for children with acute lymphocytic leukemia was only two months. But by the 1970s, chemotherapy was holding the disease in check, and 50 percent of the youngsters were living at least five years. Half of the cases of advanced Hodgkin's disease, a cancer of the lymphatic system, can now be cured with chemotherapy (and 90 percent of the early cases are arrested with radiation therapy). And for women with choriocarcinoma, a cancer involving the uterus, the statistics have changed radically with the advent of anticancer drugs: a disease that was once 90 percent fatal within a year is now 90 percent curable. The previous treatment, surgery, not only didn't work well, but it also removed the uterus and the woman's chance to have natural children — if she survived.

The use of chemotherapy has become controversial in spite of its successes because it is being pursued as a panacea for most kinds of cancers when, in fact, its effectiveness has been proven in less than 25 percent of the cancers seen clinically. The risky side effects of the drugs complicate the ethics of treatment. The drugs make the white blood count fall, increasing the patient's susceptibility to infection — a condition that could prove fatal. They also frequently damage the heart and kidneys. Hair falls out; sterility develops, either as a temporary or permanent condition; and violent nausea, cramps, and diarrhea are often common. As if all this isn't bad enough, the drugs themselves are often indicted as being cancer-producing.

Social isolation is another spin-off of chemotherapy. Just as doctors don't like to face the concept of death and terminal illness in patients, so, too, most people find it difficult to accept this state among friends. There is a lot of irrational thinking about cancer, and those suffering from it and trying to fight it with painful drugs are often avoided rather than comforted. Even well-meaning friends are afraid of "catching" cancer. One elementary school principal refused to let a child "cured" of leukemia return to her school for fear that her disease was contagious.

These virulent, vicious, and sometimes vital drugs continue to be used as ways to forestall death from cancer because, as Joseph MacDonald said, "Desperate measures must be taken for dreaded diseases."

*

Since most cancer drugs are experimental, the ethical issues involved in testing them — doing research on human subjects — have to be resolved. If doctors are to proceed ethically, they must try all other therapies before embarking on a course of treatment with experimental chemotherapies. The efficacy as well as ethics of experimenting with cancer drugs must be approved by a review board in each hospital, teaching center, or place where the drugs are dispensed. The review boards generally include physicians, hospital administrators, lawyers, ethicists, theologians, and community representatives.

The boards deal with the issue of how much benefit a patient is likely to get from the experimental drugs in comparison with the accepted conventional treatment, or how much benefit there will be to a patient with a cancer for which there is currently no treatment. "If the patient will die in two months without experimental treatment, then the risk of a drug killing him in four months is not crucial," said the chairman of a review board at a university-affiliated hospital. "But if a particular drug makes a patient more uncomfortable during his remaining days, or leaves him with horrible ulcers in his mouth so he can't eat, then the benefit of his staying alive two extra months has to be questioned, and the board would probably reject the use of that drug."

In spite of good intentions and the watchful eye of review boards, the ethics of experimenting with chemotherapy sometimes gets blurred. Are physicians treating patients or studying drugs? A standard treatment for a form of childhood leukemia, for example, involves a specific combination of drugs. The youngsters often have a relapse after treatment with this initial combination, but for some reason a second combination of experimental drugs reverses the situation and "saves" children for whom all hope was given up.

So far, so good. But one physician gave the second treatment — the experimental combination — to a fifteen-year-old girl who had not yet been given the standard treatment. The doctor's reasoning was that the experimental drugs might be able to prevent her from having a relapse. His experiment was a disaster: the drugs are probably what caused the teenager's death, even before she got a chance to try the traditional therapy.

Not all patients are good, or even proper, candidates for experimental anticancer drugs, as the case of Mrs. Luzzata illustrates. Edna Luzzata was diagnosed as having a malignant breast tumor, and had a radical mastectomy to remove it. During the course of the operation, her surgeon discovered that many lymph nodes were involved, and he removed them, too. He told Mrs. Luzzata that affected lymph nodes are often signs that the cancer will metastasize, or spread, to another part of the body. He recommended chemotherapy, since there is some promising evidence that drugs will reduce the incidence of metastases by as much as 80 percent in premenopausal women.

Mrs. Luzzata presented her physicians with a difficult ethical problem: she was two months pregnant (with her seventh child), and the toxicity risks of the drugs to a fetus were unknown. She was willing to accept the responsibility for a malformed child or a drug-induced miscarriage, but she would not have an abortion.

The cancer team debated the morality of accepting her willingness to risk her fetus's well being, and they decided to treat the patient they could see — the mother — because they felt that "this therapy was an appropriate one for her."

What Edna Luzzata did not know was that numerous cancer specialists recommended caution in using chemotherapy to prevent a recurrence of breast cancer, on the theory that drugs may suppress the immune response and may themselves cause cancer. If surgery removed all the visible cancer cells, should Mrs. Luzzata take a chance — should she even be given a chance — of exposing herself and her fetus to the risks of chemotherapy?

*

When experimental anticancer drugs are offered, most patients agree to take them. No matter how grim the side effects, for many people the certainty of death without them is grimmer. When Senator Hubert Humphrey was offered chemotherapy treatments as a way to stop his spreading cancer of the bladder, he was told that the drug was experimental. "Will it kill me or make me any worse?" asked the senator. When his physician replied no, Humphrey willingly said, "Go ahead."

Ever optimistic and ready to try something to arrest his cancer, Humphrey was told about a new possible form of cancer treatment. "It'll be just my luck," he complained. "You'll discover this cure about the time I'm ready to give up the ghost. It'll make me madder'n hell." Humphrey kept up his hopes, but lost his ten-year battle against cancer in January 1978. At his memorial service, fellow Minnesotan Vice President Walter Mondale said of Humphrey, "He taught us all how to hope and how to live, how to win and how to lose; he taught us how to live, and, finally, he taught us how to die."

Morris Abram, a noted New York lawyer and former president of Brandeis University, also had hope when he was given a diagnosis of acute myelocytic leukemia, a disease affecting the cells in the bone marrow that form white blood corpuscles. Patients have been known to die in a week to ten days after diagnosis.

"I resolved that, in my case, the disease was not going to be fatal. I was not going to give in, and I firmly resolved to defeat the disease even though I had been told by my physician that there was no hope, or very little of it."

What did he do? "I gave my permission for every kind of experimental treatment ever devised. I was desperate and determined to live," he said. And the therapy he agreed to was radical — and painful. Coupled with Abram's extraordinary determination to live was an extraordinary combination of anticancer drugs, including one that was not yet available in the United States and had to be imported from Israel. Morris Abram defied all statistics and was still alive five years later.

Not all doctors — or patients — want to pursue chemotherapy so aggressively, because of the questionable medical and moral dilemmas posed by the drugs. When Victor Billington was found to have a widespread cancer of the liver, the cancer specialist he consulted recommended series of experimental drugs in an attempt to arrest its galloping spread. His family physician, who had treated the Billingtons for fifteen years and knew Victor well, convinced him not to use any of the chemotherapies. "They couldn't do anything for GI cancers with drugs," replied the family physician. "I told him that it would be a mistake to make use of that technology. He died within three weeks of the diagnosis of liver cancer. If he had taken chemotherapy, he would have died of poisoning."

*

Danny Carter, a twenty-six-year-old newlywed, did die from the poisons of chemotherapy, according to his mother, Rose Marie Carter. "It's a form of poison," she said bitterly, several months after his death, "that is given in measured doses."

Both Beverly Carter, his widow, and Rose Marie are sorry they agreed to chemotherapy for Danny. "If we could turn back the clock to January, we would say not to go on chemotherapy," Beverly said. "But everything had to be done immediately then. Nothing was planned, and there was no time for decisions. When you're in that situation, you just don't question. Now I wish we had asked more about the disadvantages of chemotherapy."

It was in January that Danny's past history of Hodgkin's disease caught up with him. It had been treated with cobalt when he was a teen-ager, and his disease had been in remission for nearly ten years. But now it was back — and rampant.

Danny took his physicians' recommendation and began the chemotherapy treatments. He lost a lot of weight, had violent stomach cramps and spiking high temperatures. He was put in an isolation room for one week because his lowered white blood cell count, a side effect of the drugs, made him a high risk for infection. Beverly kept hoping that it was an infection that made him so sick, but it was, instead, the reaction to the chemotherapy and his spreading disease.

Over the next few months, Danny Carter became sicker and sicker. Most of his large intestine was removed, and an opening was created in his abdomen, a colostomy, connecting to his colon as an artificial passageway for excreta. He began hallucinating and had seizures because of cancerous brain lesions.

One week before he died, in late November, his brother suggested one last attempt to "get" Danny's cancer: Laetrile. "Chemotherapy had hurt him and though Laetrile might not help him, it couldn't hurt him," was Beverly's reasoning in wanting her dying husband to try this unconventional, controversial drug. "Now we wish we had looked into it earlier. But by the time Danny started treatment, his veins were too collapsed for him to get Laetrile injections, and he had to take it orally. But within a few days, it was too difficult even to get the pills into him. And then he died."

The Carters do not know what the Laetrile could have done to Danny's cancer if he had started treatments earlier, but they know what came of the chemotherapy treatments, surgery, and radiation: a lot of prolonged suffering. "It is better to take your chance with Laetrile," said his mother, "and not go through the pain."

*

The choice of drug intervention to extend life (or forestall death) in face of terminal cancer is controversial enough without adding the Laetrile issue. Is Edna Luzzata better off gambling with the health and welfare of her unborn child by taking anticancer drugs, or should she have gambled that the mastectomy had got rid of all her cancer cells? Would Morris Abram have defied the mortality statistics as he did if he had undergone a less radical drug program? Was Victor Billington's cancer too far advanced for any meaningful drug therapy to work? What does "meaningful" mean to a dying person? Less pain? Longer life in a debilitated state? A return to the normal way of living?

And now the fuzziness of Laetrile is added to all this confusion. Is Laetrile — a cyanide-bearing drug, known in pharmacology as amygdalin, that appears naturally in the pits of apricots, cherries, and other plants — a cancer cure or a quack remedy? There are more than 75,000 Americans who seek Laetrile as a cure, but it is dismissed by most medical experts in the U.S. as outright quackery and is banned by the federal government.

Which side is right? Both are, according to testimonials. A California restaurant owner with cancer of the colon refused to have the surgery his doctor recommended — removal of a bowel section and a colostomy. "Life isn't worth living like that," he said. He took vitamins, drank carrot juice, and got blood transfusions because he was so weak. When these treatments failed, he went to Mexico to a Laetrile clinic. The apricot-pit therapy seemed to work for him: his cancer subsided. But within a few months he was worse than before — "in hellish pain," he recalled — and he agreed, in desperation, to have a colostomy. The surgery appeared to be successful, but six months later he began to bleed internally and lose weight, dropping more than seventy of his normal 180 pounds. Half of his bladder was removed in an effort to root out the spreading malignancy, but surgeons could not get all the tumors. Radiation was the only alternative . . . except for Laetrile. Five years ago he decided to give it another try, and this time he "got cured." His cancer disappeared, his colostomy was reversed so that he has normal bowel function again. At fifty-nine, he feels "just fine" and is confident that the Laetrile regimen, which he is still on, has kept him alive.

When a thirty-five-year-old schoolteacher with three children was diagnosed as having cancer of the uterus in a very early stage, her doctor, too, recommended surgery. Like the restaurant owner, she refused to have the operation but began Laetrile treatments to "clear everything up without radiation or surgery or anything else." For a few months it seemed that she was getting better, but then she began bleeding and losing her strength quickly. By the time she came back to her doctor for help, the cancer had grown outside the cervix walls to the pelvis on both sides and had infiltrated the bladder to the front and the rectum to the rear. There was no longer any effective treatment available, and she died within a month.

Herein lies the kernel of the Laetrile controversy. Does a person have the right to pursue any and all treatments in an effort to live longer, or will the availability of a nonscientifically proven drug like Laetrile infringe on the patient's ability to make intelligent choices? If the schoolteacher had chosen surgery in the early stages of her cancer, there was a statistically good chance that she would still be alive. Perhaps the cancer of the restaurant owner went into a natural remission, and good luck, not Laetrile, is the reason for his present state of health.

The lack of scientific basis for decision-making further compounds the Laetrile controversy. Laboratory tests on mice consistently show Laetrile to be useless in arresting the growth of tumors. There was one exception — a preliminary study done at the Memorial Sloan-Kettering Cancer Center in New

York City, which showed that lung cancer spread in only 20 percent of the mice treated with Laetrile but spread 90 percent of the time in mice that did not receive the substance. Researchers at Sloan-Kettering and elsewhere have not been able to replicate this study or confirm its findings, and it has been dismissed as an "error."

Complicating the issue, Laetrile is now being labeled as a hazard. Cases of serious poisoning, even deaths, have been attributed to it — mostly from cyanide poisoning and microbial contamination, which causes blood poisoning, but one eleven-month-old girl died after eating five or her father's Laetrile tablets.

Though the Food and Drug Administration has banned both the approval of the drug as well as interstate shipment of it, states are beginning to give patients and physicians the right to use it. Some cancer patients get their Laetrile treatments in clinics in Mexican border towns, but most people obtain it illegally — smuggled out of Mexico, where most of it is processed. Laetrile is considered the second largest contraband imported from Mexico, after marijuana.

*

The vast array of life-extending technologies that are available gives each one of us many choices about how to die, even when to die. Having a variety of choices implies that decisions will have to be made about which one to use — and when. Dying in a technological age has become a complicated affair.

Chapter 10

Deciding to Die

A DECISION ABOUT DYING is the last important choice a person has in life. Just as there are myriads of technological interventions to postpone death, so there are myriads of decisions that are made before death can take place.

In Biblical days, Ecclesiastes preached that there is a time to die. But now choices are being made about when to die and even where to die. Treatment is refused, stopped, or sometimes never started in hopeless cases, according to the wishes of the dying patient or family members. And more people are choosing to die at home — the place where death used to take place before the advent of modern life-prolonging technologies.

There are disagreements over who has the right to make these final decisions — the patient, family, physician, hospital, or state. Each can claim the right, legally and morally.

❧A fifty-five-year-old woman has been on dialysis for eight years and decides that she no longer wants to continue treatments. Her body has rejected three kidney transplants and is not likely to accept a fourth. Dialysis is the center of her life, and it leaves her too weak and tired to do anything else.

❧Her physician agrees in principle with a patient's right to be autonomous, but his medical opinion is that she should stay on dialysis and try some new drugs to counter the side effects about which she complains.

❧The medical director of the hospital fears that if she is

allowed to stop dialysis — and therefore dies — the hospital will be liable for her death.

❡The state, meanwhile, protects individual autonomy by considering it a legal infringement on rights for doctors to give medical treatment coercively to competent adults.

This is not an isolated case of several people deciding the fate of one person's right to die. It happens often — every day, in every hospital. Sometimes all the parties agree, but more often there are clashing opinions. In spite of this state of conflict, decisions about dying must be made for many of the two million Americans who will die this year.

"No More Treatments for Me"

Sixteen-year-old Richard Greene put himself in charge of his own death when he decided during the summer not to pursue any more treatments for his rampant cancer. Earlier in the year, when his lung cancer was first detected, Richard was very optimistic about his health. "At first I felt that I could be cured," he says on a videotape he prepared just before his death, "but my cancer was so widespread that I knew it couldn't be true."

Yet Richard pursued all the vigorous courses of treatment, including chemotherapy, which made him violently ill and caused him to hallucinate. The treatments were worth the pain, he admits, because his cancer went into a remission. "I was hoping for a long-term remission — maybe I could even die of old age," he says, "but I began to get weaker and weaker, and I knew my cancer had come back."

It was difficult for Richard to decide which courses of treatment to follow for the rest of his brief life. He ruled out going to Boston or Philadelphia for special treatment because it would be impossible for his parents to travel from Connecticut, where they lived, to visit him often. And he decided not to have another round of chemotherapy injections. "It was so unpleasant before, and since it didn't work for too long, why bother going through it again if it means living only two or three more weeks? Without that treatment — or even with it — my life really can't be prolonged," says Richard realistically.

He had hoped to go back to school after the summer, but, instead, Richard went to the hospital. And he knew he went there to die. "A month ago, the x-ray showed widespread cancer in my lung. Last week it was worse, and a few days ago, even worse than that. I was told by my doctors that in two weeks it will probably be difficult for me to breathe. I am afraid of the pain of dying, and sometimes I want death to come quickly. But I can't determine the time of death. It is not up to me."

Richard died one week later. In a way, he did determine the time of his death: by accepting the harsh fact that further treatments would not help him, he refused them and thus shortened the painful and prolonged process of dying from cancer.

*

Although Richard Greene was only sixteen years old, he made a competent decision about his life and death, a decision that was supported by his parents and the hospital staff. But not everyone's wishes to terminate or refuse treatments are so readily accepted. Nor should they be. If a paranoid schizophrenic believes his food is poisoned, should he be allowed to starve to death? No, according to prevailing psychiatric opinion. It is more humane to force a patient like that to eat. Schizophrenics treated against their will are usually grateful for the help once they are better and can resume normal lives.

What happens when a mentally alert patient comes to the hospital and irrationally refuses life-saving treatment? Should physicians honor or disregard these wishes? Whose autonomy reigns?

Leonard Phillips, a forty-three-year-old accountant, was rushed by ambulance to the emergency room at the hospital.

He had severe chest pains and was having difficulty breathing — classic signs of a heart attack. The nurse was setting up a respirator to help him breathe more easily. When Phillips realized what was happening, he told the nurse, "If my heart stops beating, please don't stick all those machines on me. Let me die in peace."

Phillips had been in the hospital earlier that year, when he had had his first heart attack. During his stay on the coronary care unit, he had observed two unsuccessful attempts at resuscitation on elderly people with heart failure. He was disturbed by these efforts to prolong dying and made his doctor promise not to resuscitate him should his heart stop beating.

So here he was, back for a second round. Should his wishes not to be resuscitated be taken seriously, or had he been too frightened to make a rational statement?

Consider the opinion of Edward F. Furukawa, a physician who had had a heart attack at the age of forty-one and had been resuscitated several times during his illness. Phillips, in principle, was entitled to have a life-sustaining measure withheld if he had come to the conclusion that the quality of life which the measure gave him was not acceptable. "But," Furukawa added, "I cannot see how a patient would choose to die if he knew that his chances for survival would be very good. To allow a patient to die because he has a fear that is not clearly understood regarding treatment procedures borders on criminal negligence."

"This is not a question of ethics, but one of psychology," said Harvard psychiatrist Avery Weisman, commenting on the case. "Despair can be fleeting, and in the morning, this man might have felt quite differently about himself and his future."

Leonard Phillips was resuscitated by the nurse in the emergency room, but when Phillips's physician came — the one with whom he made the deal "not to resuscitate" — all life-saving measures were stopped. Phillips died a half hour later.

*

Fern Terry, a sixty-one-year-old woman suffering from a brain tumor, was once as frightened about having radiation treatment as was Phillips about being resuscitated. But rather than accept her negative feelings — uttered at a time when she was of sound mind but nonetheless depressed and in great pain — her physician, family, and friends tried to reason with her. Fern Terry eventually changed her mind, began radiation treatments, and took a longer lease on life to get some extra time to spend with her husband, George, in their new retirement home, built with an indoor swimming pool on top of a hill overlooking ten acres of rich farmland in the rolling Maryland countryside.

The Terrys moved to their dream home in September, but Fern had very bad headaches and was never well enough to enjoy it. "We always thought these temporary ailments would pass away," recalled her husband, "but this one did not." By Christmas she was in great pain, and in February a large tumor was detected on the right side of her brain by the CAT scanner. Part of the tumor was removed — it was too large and deep to be taken out entirely — but the doctors recommended radiation treatments as a way to erode many of the remaining cancer cells.

Fern adamantly refused. Her sister had died five years before, after she was exposed to cobalt treatments to arrest an abdominal cancer. The cobalt treatments had indeed stopped the growth of her sister's cancer, but it had also destroyed other tissues — specifically, it had weakened her intestines.

"When her sister died, her cancer had been eradicated, but it was the cobalt that did her in. My wife had this memory in mind," said George Terry, "and she made me promise not to subject her to cobalt — just to let her die quietly. She talked a lot about dying — about what songs she wanted sung at her memorial service, what to do with her clothes and jewelry. She even suggested who would make me a good second wife."

No one could force Fern to change her mind. The decision was hers to make, keep, or change. Her doctor told her that though radiation treatments wouldn't cure her cancer, they would likely extend her life. As one example, he told her about a patient with a similar brain tumor who was alive and active at the time, eight years after treatment.

From being adamant — absolutely no radiation — Fern slowly began to reconsider. She was in less pain than when she had initially refused radiation treatment, because the pressure of the tumor on her brain had been relieved by surgery. The stories her doctor told her sounded encouraging, even enticing. But what finally made her change her mind was being greeted, when she came home from the hospital, by her three children and five grandchildren, ranging in age from six months to ten years. She couldn't bear the thought of not living to see the grandchildren grow up.

Once Fern Terry changed her mind and wanted radiation treatments, she also added chemotherapy to the roster of things that might help extend her life. She was in great discomfort as a result of her decision: the radiation burned her scalp, and the chemotherapy made her nauseated. But she desperately wanted to try to live longer.

Fern Terry gambled but lost. She died barely six months after she had had the radiation treatments to wipe out her cancer.

Fighting Medical Decisions in Court

George Terry, Fern's doctor, and even the grandchildren were all part of an attempt to get Fern to change her mind about refusing radiation treatments, but there was nothing morally, legally, or medically wrong with her not having them. Numerous court proceedings have supported a competent patient's right to refuse treatment, based on the principle of freedom and self-determination. "It is the individual who is the subject of a medical decision who has the final say," ruled one judge.

The right to refuse treatment becomes an ethical issue when the patient is mentally or physically incompetent to make that decision by him or herself, when children are involved, and when it does not adhere to sound medical practice.

When Delores and Bob Sutter's second child was born, they were horrified to find out that she had spina bifida. The physician told the shocked Sutters about the disease and its possible outcome, and stressed that for Sondra the outcome looked very good — if she had surgery to close the opening in her spine and to put in a shunt to drain the fluid collecting in her head. If the spine remained open it could become seriously infected, and if the shunt were not put in irreversible brain damage could develop.

"The parents stalled in making the decision whether or not to treat," recalled the neurosurgeon in charge of the case, Dr. David McCullough. "They said they didn't have enough information on which to make a decision, even though we spent more than six hours with them explaining the situation and giving them literature to read about it. We gave them as much information as was available. But we couldn't tell them what their child would be like at the age of seventy-two. I can't even tell what *I'll* be like at seventy-two," said McCullough, now in his mid-forties.

Parents generally accept suggestions by physicians about treatment of deformed newborns. They treat if a physician suggests it, and they don't treat when a physician thinks that is best. But cases occasionally arise where there is a disagreement, and parents refuse to treat a youngster who, by medical criteria, will have a good outcome. Such was the case with the Sutters.

"We couldn't accept the parents' indecision. They were delaying, and this was dangerous for the baby," Dr. McCullough said. "The well-being of the child was being compromised, and we had to step in."

The case went to court, Sondra became a ward of the state, and her parents abdicated all responsibilities. The opening in her spine was closed and a shunt inserted. Sondra is now three years old — a beautiful, happy child, of normal intelligence, walking well with leg braces and living in a permanent foster home. She has not seen her parents again, nor is she ever likely to see them.

The Teagues also faced a court fight over not treating their spina bifida baby, Samantha, but it was an ugly, vindictive fight, based not on medical principles but on the ethics of the custodial physician. Kay and Michael Teague, a young British couple living in Maryland, have talked openly about the event — the birth, brief life, and death of their daughter.

When Samantha was born in the early fall, Kay sensed something was wrong because the doctor didn't say, "It's a boy" or "It's a girl." He just gasped. Michael, an aeronautical physicist who was attending the natural delivery, blurted out, "Oh my God, what's wrong with her legs?" and then passed out. Michael woke up in the emergency room, where he was x-rayed for a fractured skull and monitored for a possible heart attack. All he had broken was his glasses, but he remained in shock for a while.

The cause of his shock was Samantha's condition. She was born with a large opening high on her spine and grossly deformed legs, which went up to her face from the waist instead of straight down. Her knees bent the wrong way, and her feet were clubbed.

"She has a hole in her back that can be closed up," explained the pediatrician to the Teagues, "but she will be left with some paralysis." Kay was stunned, but followed the doctor's suggestion to have Samantha transferred to Children's Hospital, where she would have surgery. "Of course we wanted to have corrective surgery on Samantha," said Kay, "given the information we had."

But there was a series of events that changed the situation. A neurosurgeon came to examine Samantha to see if the surgery was warranted. When Kay heard this, she was very confused. If the neurosurgeon was questioning Samantha's condition, then it was possible that no surgery would be in order. And if that was the case, then Samantha's case was hopeless.

And this is just what happened. The neurosurgeon recommended no treatment. He predicted that she would live less than six months without surgery, and that with surgery she was likely to live four or five years, with one painful surgical experience after another, paralyzed, retarded, in the hospital more than she would be out of it. The Teagues sought the opinion of other surgeons and had this grim prognosis confirmed.

Kay and Michael agreed that they would each make an independent decision, but that if either one of them decided to go ahead with the surgery, the other would agree to it. While they were making their decisions, Samantha's head size grew substantially. The 85 percent chance of her getting hydrocephalus was confirmed.

"We both decided not to treat. She would not live long no matter what we did," Kay said. "We could prolong her life, but it would be at a great discomfort to her. When you make a decision to have children, you have to decide to do what is best for that child. We made this decision for Samantha — not for us."

Kay and Michael wanted Samantha to come home, but they were advised against it. It would have been difficult for Sean (a son who was then three years old), and impossible to keep things sterile. Instead, they placed her in a state institution for mentally retarded children, and here is where their troubles began. The chief medical officer thought that Samantha should be treated surgically, whether her prognosis was poor or not, "and she wanted to get her way," Kay recalled bitterly.

She almost did — but for a fluke intervention. "One day while we were visiting Samantha, we stopped at the nursing station to find out what foods she was eating, and the nurse told us, 'She can't eat tonight because she is scheduled for

surgery tomorrow morning at seven-thirty.' Just like that" —
Kay snapped her fingers — "we found out about a plan we
specifically said we did not want."

The surgeon who was scheduled to perform the operation
had been led to believe that Samantha was a ward of the
state and that he had carte blanche to do the surgery. "He
was shocked to find out that we disagreed with the principle
of surgery for Samantha," added Kay.

Legally and morally, he could not go through with the
operation, even though he thought that Samantha should
have it, but he did raise some serious questions for the
Teagues by giving a new prognosis. Samantha, he said, *might*
be able to walk — no one before had intimated that there
was a remote possibility of her walking — and that there was
a reasonable chance that she would have a normal intelligence.

Samantha was now six weeks old. The Teagues had already
made one decision about her, based on one prognosis. Now
they would have to make another decision, based on a second
prognosis. They thought it over, consulted more physicians,
and came to the conclusion that the second prognosis was
not realistic and that it was a justification for the surgeon's
ethics. The staff at the state institution were instructed to
give Samantha only palliative care — no heroics.

In early December, the Teagues were brought to court in
a dramatic attempt by the state to get temporary medical
custody of Samantha to close the spinal lesion, surgically reconstruct her legs, and perform a shunt operation. The first
two procedures were subsequently dropped from the charge
because it was not crucial to do them at that time. But without the shunt operation, argued officials from the state institution, Samantha would not live more than two days.

The judge felt that each party was doing what it thought
was in the best interests of the patient, but that since the
request for surgery was not based on a definitive, uncontested
recommendation and since there were conflicting medical

opinions about treatment, it was not a question for the law to handle.

Before the judge had a chance to make a decision, a woman from the state institution rushed into the courtroom with the news that Samantha had taken a turn for the worse. The case was withdrawn.

Meanwhile, back at the state institution, nurses were ordered to place Samantha in an oxygen tent, even though the Teagues had requested "no heroics." "They put her there to prolong her life — even when she was on her way out of it," said Kay angrily. Samantha died two days later.

"Even if the state had been successful in getting permission to do the surgery," Michael said, "the timing was ludicrous. She was dying at the point that they wanted to operate. If she was to be treated, it should have been in the first few days of her life. The law can't move fast enough for medical events like this.

"Parents are the ones who should make the decisions about their children's care. But some checks and balances are needed since some parents go against uncontested medical opinion [as did the Sutters], and there is a need for the state to intervene when the parents aren't acting in the best interests of the child. In Samantha's case, what the state wanted to do would not have helped her."

Who makes the decision about whether the state should intervene, and whether or not the parents are acting in the best interests of the child? Because of the way Samantha resolved the case — by dying — the questions remain moot.

When the Time Comes

"I don't think I want life-extending facilities for Jeff," commented Carolyn Sinclair, whose twelve-year-old son has been sick from birth. "But I may change my mind when the time comes."

Jeffrey inherited a rare disease, Hunter's syndrome, which results in stunted growth, both mentally and physically, and abnormalities in the heart and lung. (The genetic history of Jeffrey Sinclair's condition is discussed in Chapter 2.) Doctors predict a life span of ten to fifteen years for Jeff, so he is nearing the end — and his mother is trying to prepare for it. He has a severe leak in the aortic valve in his heart, his respiratory tract is constantly inflamed so it is hard for him to breathe, and he finds it difficult to swallow most foods. He already has had one stroke and is likely to have more.

Jeffrey spends weekdays at a state school for the mentally handicapped and comes home on weekends to be with his mother and younger brother, Christopher. Carolyn is considering putting Jeff at school as a full boarder when his condition deteriorates further — "when he no longer recognizes me and Chris." She does not know when that state of deterioration will come — three months? three years? — but she knows that it will come.

"I have protected Jeff all of his life, and always will," she said, "but when he really deteriorates there would be no point in trying to extend his life. He has suffered enough. Anyway, extending his life won't change the course of his disease. It might be different if there was a chance that he could benefit from a cure if he were kept alive longer, but that's not possible. The most it can do is keep him with me a little longer, and that would be at his expense."

Although Carolyn Sinclair has given a lot of thought to the meaning of Jeffrey's life and death, she cautioned, "I am not foolish enough to think that the decision about using or not using things to extend his life will be easy when the time comes."

*

The decision to start — or stop — life-support or last-ditch measures of any sort is never easy. Although Carolyn has had a long time to prepare for Jeffrey's death, she is still unsure how she will react at the end. The Browns had no time to prepare their thoughts about death when forty-five-year-old Francis Brown collapsed without any warning at his office one day with a massive cerebral hemorrhage. The Brown family was in a state of shock, unable to comprehend the gravity of the situation even when he was placed on a respirator. The physician, however, knew the seriousness of his condition and that death was likely.

Twenty-four hours after Brown's admission to the hospital, the family began to become aware of his poor prognosis. The idea of discontinuing the respirator was aired by various physicians and nurses on the ICU, but the family wanted to wait another twenty-four hours to re-evaluate his condition.

Forty-eight hours made it more clear that his death was imminent. Francis Brown showed no signs of improvement or of triggering the respirator on his own, yet his seventeen-year-old son, Brian, was still not ready to "disconnect Daddy's machine." Brian was ready to accept the inevitable the next day, three days after his father's fatal stroke. "It was time," he said, acknowledging that *he* needed the time to accept the fact of death. Francis Brown died eighteen minutes after the respirator was disconnected. He made no attempts to breathe. His heart stopped. The time had come.

*

When twenty-nine-year-old John Schuler's time had come, no one in the family wanted to believe it either — even though he had been sickly throughout his life, trying to fight off respiratory diseases as a result of his cystic fibrosis. His family considered John "well," since he suffered only from chronic bronchitis, in contrast to his younger sister, who died at fifteen from pulmonary complications of cystic fibrosis.

For the last two years of his life, John Schuler was on a downhill course. The bronchitis developed into the more serious and ultimately fatal condition called bronchiectasis, in which mucus builds up in the lungs. He took a variety of antibiotics, becoming immune to one after the other, and an experimental drug that left him vulnerable to blood diseases, so he had to have blood samples taken every ten days. John also developed painful neuritis in his feet, lost part of his hearing, and expelled a very bad odor from the mucus in his lung.

Lorraine, his wife, was his cheerleader. "I wouldn't let him talk about dying," she said. "It was bad enough for him to drag himself around with that bad cough, crummy pain in his feet, and bad smell without having the burden of thinking he was going to die, too."

John went to the hospital every few months, mostly to have the excess mucus removed from his lungs. He usually felt great after this procedure, but the ninth time he went in, the procedure didn't work. Not enough of the mucus could be removed, and the remaining thick layers of it severely compromised his breathing. One lung collapsed, and he was rushed to the intensive care unit, where he was put on a respirator and closely monitored. He remained there for three weeks — weak, tired, and with low morale. He tried, but could not wean himself from the respirator. The doctors knew that John was dying and that there was nothing else they could do to save his life. They could only prolong it.

Lorraine could not accept this; it took away her hope. "I knew he was in bad trouble, but I did not believe he would die — until the day he actually did," she confessed. "I was waiting to take him home with me, but if he had come home, he would have been tied to an oxygen machine, and it would have killed him inside. I would have taken him in any condition, I wanted him so badly. But the medical people are really better judges. They don't have this kind of attachment.

"The day he died, he looked as if he was sleeping, but he was so white. That was when I knew the doctors were right and I was wrong: John was really dying. He hated being sick," Lorraine said softly, "but his dying was meant to be." Lorraine gave the orders to let nature take its course.

Alternative Deathstyles

To avoid deathbed disappointments, difficult decision-making about when and how to stop prolonging death, as well as the indignities and inconsistencies of the aggressive "therapeutic" treatment dying patients in hospitals often endure, more and more people are choosing to die at home — free from medical interventions.

When Senator Philip Hart, of Michigan, lay dying of cancer in 1976, he did it quietly, with his wife, Jane, and his eight children surrounding him twenty-four hours a day with love and care in his family home in Washington, D.C. A downstairs room was fitted with a hospital bed for him and a single bed for the person who spent the night with him. Each night a different family member slept in the bed next to the dying Senator — to care for him, to watch over him. The Hart family fed him, bathed him, gave him painkilling injections, which made him reasonably comfortable though somewhat disoriented at times. "He won't be going to the hospital," said his wife during the final stages of his illness. And he didn't. He died in control of his death, at home, without medical meddling.

*

"When you're in patients' homes, in contrast to being in a hospital, you're on their territory, and you can't tell them what to do," observed Alise Green, the nurse of the home-care cancer program at the Georgetown University Hospital. "At home, the dying patient is in control."

There are currently twenty patients in the Georgetown home-care program, and each patient is dying of cancer in spite of previous attempts to "cure" the disease with the traditional anticancer treatments — surgery, radiation, and chemotherapy. There are no more treatments to try. All they need is loving helpers to feed and bathe them, to administer pain medication, and to try to protect them from the loneliness of dying.

The members of the home-care team — a nurse, a social worker, and a physician — give emotional support, pain medication, and professional advice. They do anything to help make the final weeks or months of life comfortable, but they no longer give treatments to prolong life.

"We don't give drugs to help them with their appetite or push food in them through tubes," said Dr. Peter Petrucci. "Instead, we give them supportive therapy, such as 'You need to eat to keep up your strength.'" The average home-care patient keeps up his or her strength for two to three months before dying at home.

Contrast this to a hospital, where there is a tendency for the staff to "do more" in an attempt to help the dying, even though aggressive treatments to prolong living can no longer prevent death. "Sometimes dying patients are put on respirators in hospitals to clear up difficulties in breathing," said Alise Green. "But this is unrealistic because, as a person dies, breathing naturally becomes irregular.

"Hospitals are acute-care settings, and few nurses are trained for chronic care, which is the kind of care terminal cancer patients need. If 'no code' is written on the charts — the medical profession's shorthand for 'do not resuscitate' — then the patient often gets neglected by the hospital staff in the mistaken belief that they are to leave the patient alone to die. However, if no notation is made, then it often means that things will be done to extend unnecessarily the life of a dying person."

*

The dying days of sixty-five-year-old Mary Willis are spent in a hospital bed in the living room of a small, one-bedroom apartment she has shared with her boyfriend, Douglas Argent, for several years. ("I had three bad marriages," she said on one of her more lucid days, "and did not want to gamble on a fourth.") It is dark in the apartment where she lies, moribund. She is semicomatose, no longer talking, but occasionally she opens her eyes. Her breathing is noisy. Attentive to the signs of the terminally ill, Alise Green tells Dougie that this breathing is often called the death rattle.

Mary Willis had fought against cancer when she was a young woman; twenty-five years ago she had breast cancer but, with a radical mastectomy, she had licked it. She wasn't as lucky the second time around, and now she is dying of a brain tumor. Half of the tumor was removed by surgery, but the remainder was not responsive to radiation or drug treatments.

While she was still thinking and talking clearly, she made her dying wishes known: she refused to go back on chemotherapy, and she refused to return to the hospital. Mary wanted to die at home, with Dougie. He kisses her and grieves. He calls her and waits for an answer. "She hasn't talked to me in so long," he says quietly, "but this morning she opened her eyes and looked at me."

Dougie waits on Mary. He meticulously crushes fruit cocktail for her to eat, although all she may eat in a day is a few teaspoons. He paints her fingernails and toenails, and rubs her feet to reduce swelling. He reads mail from relatives to her ("Please tell Grandma," wrote an eight-year-old grandson in Texas, "that I made $2 pulling weeds"). And he always sleeps in the green plastic chair by her bedside, holding her hand. Just two weeks ago he could take her out in her wheelchair, but now she lies virtually lifeless.

Dougie knows that Mary is dying. "Even with your help she will die. But you're doing a good job," Alise Green reassures him. "Mary is where she wanted to be, and is getting good care."

He nods slowly. "Yeah, she hated being in that hospital. She told me — the last time she talked — 'Don't leave me.' Like I would ever leave her." And he weeps. As painful as this is for Dougie, Mary is spending her final days, perhaps her final hours, immersed in love and affection, dying at home, without technological interventions.

Interest in dying at home is swelling throughout the U.S. There are more than fifty home-care programs for the dying across the country, including special programs for children with terminal illness for whom there is no longer any medical help or hope.

Home care was what Mary Willis wanted, what Phil Hart wanted — but it is not what everyone wants. A thirty-eight-year-old man with head and face cancer tried it, but quickly returned to the hospital. Half of his face was eroded away, and it was ugly and had a bad odor. He had four young children at home, and his condition was too unpleasant and difficult for them to cope with.

In another situation, a man with liver cancer wanted to die at home, and his wife thought she could manage the care that he needed. But when he became terminal, she panicked. Who would declare him dead? How would his body be removed? When he became comatose, she got hysterical. The physician was caught in the middle. Which was he supposed to satisfy — the wife's anxiety or the husband's wish to die at home? The patient died six hours later, in the hospital. "I did what was best not for my patient but for his wife," explained the physician. "These kinds of medical ethics issues are more important than whether or not to pull the plug on someone who is already brain-dead."

For some dying patients, home care is not the answer because there is no one there to do the caring. Fifty-five-year-old Gabriel Oleaga came to the hospital with advanced cancer of the pancreas. There were no more treatments for him, but he came and stayed a week because he had severe abdominal pain. He returned to the hospital two days after he left, with complaints of nausea and severe bouts of vomiting. After another week's stay in the hospital, he went home. This routine continued, and on his fourth admission to the hospital Mrs. Oleaga said, "Please let my husband stay in the hospital. I have used up my vacation time and have to return to work. We have no children and no one to care for him at home. He will be all alone and frightened if he stays at home."

*

A solution for patients like Gabriel Oleaga is a hospital-like setting for the terminally ill — in a hospice, or way station for travelers; in this case, for people traveling to the end of their lives. A hospice can provide what hospitals fail to give — personalized attention, care, and compassion for the very special needs of the dying patient and the patient's family.

There are several hospices providing this kind of care, but the best known is St. Christopher's Hospice in London — run by the dynamic Dr. Cicely Saunders, who for more than a decade has been helping people there during the final few days and weeks of their lives. St. Christopher's has been described as "a place to go when the doctor says there is no more to be done." "It's not like a hospital," said one patient; "it's more like a big parlor." "A kind of convalescent home — no, more like a family," said another.

St. Christopher's has no sophisticated resuscitation equipment, because, as Dr. Saunders said, "we do not treat acute remedial patients. We might resuscitate staff or visitors, which we have done on occasion, but mainly we treat irremedial illness." Even though there is no aggressive treatment for these patients, Saunders emphasized, "we certainly do all we can to fulfill a patient's potential for living well until he dies."

This includes a regimen of complete pain control, thus eliminating some of the most debilitating and dehumanizing aspects of terminal cancer. St. Christopher's specializes in a heroin cocktail, a successful and controversial method of pain control. There are visitors at St. Christopher's at all times of the day and night, and children are allowed — indeed, encouraged — to come, too. Since the staff members spend no time trying to administer life-saving measures, they have more time to listen to the wishes and fears, hopes and desires, of their dying patients. All of this for approximately one-third to one-half the cost of a modern hospital, with its array of life-saving equipment — so unnecessary for these patients.

Hospice, Inc., in New Haven, Connecticut (one of the best in the U.S.), is modeling itself after St. Christopher's, with both home care and a hospice facility; and in Washington, D.C., a portion of an unused floor in a home for incurable patients was converted into a hospice. There are 20,000 nursing homes in the U.S., many of which can be redesigned, with creative thinking, to accommodate a hospice wing. It is predicted that hospice facilities will expand, as the needs of the dying become more apparent, and as more people decide to assert their autonomy and die as naturally as possible — without technological interventions.

Chapter 11

Pulling the Plug

IN THE surgical and burn intensive care unit of a major metropolitan hospital, three patients were dying. They were adults who had no chance of emerging from their comatose states, yet they lay there, consuming hundreds of thousands of dollars' worth of medical equipment and around-the-clock medical care because no one was willing to make the decision to let them die.

The first patient, seventy-year-old Donald Watkins, had been found when the police entered his apartment after the neighbors noticed that he had not "been around" for several days. Watkins, a senile man with no known family, was suffering from what was first diagnosed as a perforated ulcer, a curable and easily operable condition. But when surgery was performed, a perforated cancer of the stomach was detected — a condition that, his surgeon said, "has a miserable outcome."

Donald Watkins never fully awoke from his operation. He was unconscious but had reflexes, such as blinking and swallowing. He had been in the intensive care unit for six weeks and likely would have remained there, since no one was willing to make a decision to give him less than full treatment. But fate changed his destiny when a woman with a severe infection in her bile ducts came into the unit. "If we pulled her through," said a surgeon on the unit, "she would be able to go home and lead a normal, full life."

To make room for her, Mr. Watkins, Patient One, was

triaged — transferred from the unit to a regular hospital ward, where he was neither as aggressively treated nor as intensively observed. The chances that he would die there, in contrast to the ICU, were vastly increased.

A decision — by default — was made about Patient One. Donald Watkins died eight days after he left the intensive care unit.

The second patient on the unit, a sixty-five-year-old woman, came in with burns over 25 percent of her body. Although Laura Lipschultz was in pain, she was talking and joking about how she finally got caught smoking in bed. A skin graft was performed on her immediately, to help the healing process and to deter infection. But soon after the operation she had a cardiac arrest — her heart stopped beating.

Mrs. Lipschultz was revived and placed on a respirator in an attempt to stabilize her condition, but it only worsened. She had repeated heart failures; her burns became infected; her body was septic and full of pus; and the grafts did not take. Complicating the matter, she was diabetic; her condition was difficult to control; she went into insulin shock and eventually a coma. She did not have a flat EEG, but she also did not show any prospects of improving. Mrs. Lipschultz had a devoted family, but after she had been in a coma for two weeks, her children asked the staff to "please let her die."

The ICU staff made no decision about Patient Two. "She died of her own accord a month after her accident," said one of the attending physicians on the unit, "but you could not really say she died naturally."

The third patient, sixty-eight-year-old Walden Asbury, was an old-timer on the ICU. He had come in nearly half a year before with a stroke and with burns over 45 percent of his body. It was never clear which came first, the stroke or the burns. Did he have a stroke and therefore get caught in a fire, or did he get caught in a fire and then have a stroke?

It is a moot point — one Asbury was never able to clear up, because all he did was lie in bed, as he had ever since he entered the hospital, and grunt. He was awake, but barely, and no one knew if he comprehended anything that was going on around him. He could breathe solely with the help of a mechanical respirator. His only relatives, distant cousins, gave up visiting him or even inquiring about him soon after he entered the hospital.

Mr. Asbury had, and caused, many problems during this time. His flesh was eroded down to the bone on his fingers. One eye was blinded by burn-related infections, and the other was seriously injured. Although he was too septic and infected for his grafts to take, attempts were repeatedly made, and he used up much of the limited supplies of cadaver skin. He also had repeated cardiac arrests.

Asbury's infections and recurring pneumonia were treated initially with antibiotics, but he eventually became resistant to all the drugs given to him and began colonizing untreatable bacteria. One of his "roommates," a man with burns over 30 percent of his body and a good chance of recovery, caught a drug-resistant infection from Asbury and died. Walden Asbury was put in isolation — in a sterile room by himself, to protect the other patients. Since this hospital has only four-bed rooms, no singles, he deprived three other patients of the chance to receive the special care given in the ICU.

"There he was — suffering, harmful to the other patients, occupying a vitally needed room, using costly and limited supplies," said an attending physician, "and even if everything went right, he was a functionless human being, and would remain a functionless human being."

Why did this treatment continue? Because no one was willing to make a decision to let him die.

There were three physicians assigned to the intensive care unit. One came to the decision, after Mr. Asbury had been in the hospital for three months, that it was not worth prolonging his inevitable death. The second physician used all the tricks in his burn-specialist bag and, though none worked, he didn't want to give up trying to have the grafts take. The

third and senior physician believed that the next sophisticated lab test would uncover the mystery of Asbury's infections. And so he ordered more and more lab tests and
treated Asbury aggressively on the basis of the test findings.
Blood tests, cultures, x-rays — if something was out of kilter,
Asbury got transfusions, drugs, extra nutrition, anything, in a
desperate attempt to keep him alive.

Without aggressive treatment, Walden Asbury surely
would have died. His pneumonia would have gotten worse,
and he would have become more septic and infected. But
aggressive treatments for Mr. Asbury continued.

"How could we kill a patient?" asked one of the three ICU
physicians. "We couldn't put a scalpel in his heart. 'Don't
use heroic means' is nice terminology, but what does it mean?
Don't pump on his chest if he has a cardiac arrest? Don't
give antibiotics? Where is the line between heroic and
ordinary?"

Patient Three died by another default decision: when the
most aggressive treater went on vacation, Walden Asbury began receiving palliative, not life-extending, care. He was given
liquids to make him comfortable, not supernutrition to make
him stronger. He died, on the respirator, less than two weeks
later.

"We didn't play God with these three patients," one of the
ICU doctors made clear. "Intervening when God obviously
wants a patient to die is not playing God."

For Donald Watkins, Laura Lipschultz, and Walden Asbury, decisions about their appropriate care and appropriate
deaths were never rationally formulated. Each death was prolonged and occurred finally, in spite of the fact that no one decided when to let it happen mercifully.

The hospital in which these three deaths took place is not
unique in its lack of rules or guidance for treating dying patients. Although at least 80 percent of physicians across the
country have at some time stopped trying to prolong the life
of a patient, there are few guidelines for discharging this awesome responsibility.

Order Out of Chaos: Hospital Guidelines for the Dying

"Do everything you can, but if the patient arrests, do not resuscitate" is a common but contradictory hospital order that means everyone has given up on the patient but does not have enough nerve to say quit.

In New York City's Mount Sinai Hospital, in the Falk Surgical-Respiratory Intensive Care Unit, conflicting orders no longer exist. Instead, there is a rational decision-making process that establishes four levels of care — from all-out therapeutic efforts to the discontinuation of therapy and life-supports. The category system was designed to alleviate the ambiguities involved in determining whether a person is in a hopeless state or a viable state, and what constitutes appropriate care.

"If a patient is worth working on," explained Dr. Christopher Bryan-Brown, the British-born director of the unit, "the only way to work on him is flat out. If there's even a small chance, give him full support — but don't give just enough support to let him die slowly. We no longer accept a policy that permits us to give patients an antibiotic for an infection but not a transfusion if they are bleeding. A patient is worth treating outright — or not at all. Half-treatment is a terrible way to let a patient die."

Since 1972, every one of the 700 to 1000 patients coming to the eighteen-bed Falk ICU each year is automatically placed in Category I, all-out therapy, until his or her case is evaluated according to the plan set up by the former ICU director, Garth Tagge; the present director, Bryan-Brown; and nurse-clinician Diane Adler. Most of the patients remain in Category I and eventually become well enough to leave the hospital. But about 15 percent of the patients admitted each year die; they are too sick to recover.

Patients are moved to Category II when there is still a chance of survival — though a remote one — even if they have not improved with the all-out efforts. They receive the same treatment as in Category I, but their prognosis is re-evaluated every twelve to twenty-four hours. If they start to improve, they move back to Category I, but if their prognosis worsens, they may move down to the next step.

When there is no measurable chance of survival, patients are put in Category III. No treatment is initiated there. Patients receive conservative, passive care — comfort measures only, with no heroics to preserve life. They do not receive blood transfusions if they hemorrhage; they are not given antibiotics if infections develop. And they are not resuscitated if they have cardiac arrest. If a patient was placed on a respirator or outfitted with intravenous tubes for feeding before entering Category III, however, this support is not withdrawn.

"Those given comfort measures only [in Category III] have some vital signs but are not conscious," Dr. Bryan-Brown explained. "Everything else we tried has failed. If we are not applying treatments which don't work anyway, then we are not doing anything different in terms of the patient's outcome."

Karen Ann Quinlan, as well as the three patients described on the burn-surgical ICU — Donald Watkins, Laura Lipschultz, and Walden Asbury — would probably have been placed in Category III, once hope for their recovery was abandoned. Without aggressive treatment, they might have died in a fairly short time.

Virtually every patient placed in Category III has died — with the exception of two "miracle" patients, who moved from "comfort measures only" right on up until they walked out of the hospital. Each of these recoveries was so spectacular that everyone on the unit hopes another will happen.

Category IV is for the brain-dead. All therapy and life-support assistance are discontinued. "Patients with cerebral death do not cause us problems," said Dr. Bryan-Brown, "because there are methods for determining brain death pretty well." Mount Sinai has officially adopted the Harvard criteria for brain death, which includes two flat electroencephalograph readings, twenty-four hours apart.

"But problems arise when a patient isn't brain-dead," the ICU director continued. "We physicians are being asked to do too much. The categories were set up because we were busting ourselves to get someone better who did not have a hope of survival. We were told to 'do everything you can,' and then were left with a hopeless case." With the classification system, no one has to "do everything" for the 4 percent of patients on whom all-out efforts are halted each year.

When the medical team decides that there is nothing more that can be done, this decision is explained to the family. "We do not put them [the family] in a position of having to make a decision, but we ask if they would like to have an outside medical consultant, so if they object they have an alternative to pursue," Dr. Bryan-Brown said.

Most families do not insist on keeping a patient alive as long as possible. Conversely, the more common problem is that the family wants to give up when the medical staff still believes that there is hope.

Consider the example of the eighty-year-old woman — the mother of a physician — who came into the ICU after an operation to amputate her foot because of a vascular disease. She had a poor recovery from the operation, and suffered a heart attack. The ICU staff did not question her ability to get well, but her son was adamant about not having her resuscitated if she had another heart attack. "She has led a good and long life," he reasoned. "Why have her suffer as an invalid?"

The staff persisted in treating her aggressively because it thought that was the only sound medical decision and was also in her own best interests. When she went home from the hospital, she was walking steadily with a cane and on a prosthesis, and she lived comfortably for eighteen months before she died of further complications of her vascular disease.

The system at Mount Sinai provides a reasonably open forum on the course of treatment and tends to eliminate the kind of staff conflict that surrounded the care and eventual death of Walden Asbury. Too many patients like Mr. Asbury have been treated aggressively during their dying days because a physician or nurse refused to "let that patient die on my shift." The dying patient will die anyway, but the Mount Sinai system allows the patient to have appropriate care, rather than a prolonged affair because no one could agree on what was appropriate.

*

Determining prognosis is an essential step in arriving at an appropriate decision about the treatment of dying patients, but it is only a first step. Hospitals across the country are exploring different solutions to problems raised by the need to make those decisions — from hospital ethical review committees to patient autonomy. None of these systems is perfect, but all represent an attempt to grapple with a difficult issue and a trend toward treating the dying more humanely and with dignity.

When staff physicians at the Massachusetts General Hospital in Boston became increasingly concerned, in 1973, that intensive care units were overdoing it — perhaps even abusing some dying patients with overzealous treatment — a Critical Care Committee was set up. A patient-classification system similar to the Mount Sinai categories was established, as well as an Optimum Care Committee to serve in an advisory capacity "in situations where difficulties arise in deciding the appropriateness of continuing intensive therapy for critically ill patients." The special advisory committee includes six specialists — a surgeon, an internist, a nun-nurse, a Jesuit priest–psychiatrist, a hospital attorney, and a former patient (a woman who had survived a rare sarcoma from which all other persons known to have the disease died). They do not make judgments on the merits of the case of each dying patient, but rather they are called on as consultants for difficult cases, and only when the physician in charge requests their help.

Typical of the cases on which they counsel is a conflict among staff members: a physician wants to continue aggressive treatment on a man with brain damage, liver failure, and repetitive cardiac arrests, because he feels that the patient is not beyond hope. The nursing staff argues that the patient's brain is barely active and that continuing care for him is inhumane and undignified, as well as a waste of time and money. The committee reviews the nature and extent of his illness and what, if anything, can be done to restore health to the patient.

"For most of these people," said Ned Cassem, the priest-psychiatrist who serves as chairman of the Optimum Care Committee, "life has already been taken away because of the disease process. Our concern is humane intervention into that process. Just because we have the technology does not mean we are obliged to use it."

The Massachusetts General committee has resolved nearly two dozen conflicts about ICUs during its first three years, but it has been criticized for focusing on the relationship between the physician and the hospital staff, with little regard to the rights of the patients and their families.

*

An approach to the dilemma of dying that requires patient or family consent is being tested by Beth Israel Hospital, also in Boston — ironically, the same city where the medical intrusion on the sanctity of life was questioned over abortion in the Edelin case. The idea for Beth Israel's Orders Not to Resuscitate (ONTR) developed after the director of the hospital, Mitchell Rabkin, was walking down the corridor and saw a nurse standing outside a patient's room, weeping. "Why can't they let him die in peace?" she asked Dr. Rabkin. The nurse had been taking care of a man with metastatic lung cancer. He was in great pain, short of breath, and had just suffered a cardiac arrest. Someone had rung the bell for immediate help, and the medical staff, which is geared to save patients' lives and respond to the hospitalwide alarm of cardiac arrest, was in the room, resuscitating him.

"This exemplifies the dilemma we face," explained Dr. Rabkin. "It is a procedural dilemma. The hospital must be pro-life. When you see someone who looks as if he is dying, you don't question whether it is moral or ethical to save him. You just go. When the alarm rings in the fire station, firemen don't question whether to go or not. They just go."

For dying patients, however a pro-life approach and the continuation of life-supporting care can be abusive. The nurse at Beth Israel had lavished efforts on her patient to let him die in peace. He was almost there, and now everything she and the patient worked for was being reversed, and the patient's dying process was forestalled.

Dr. Rabkin thought about this incident — clearly not an isolated one in his or any other hospital — and decided that there was a need for a system that recognized the patient's right to die. Beth Israel had previously shown its concern for patients by being the first hospital in the country to draw up a patient's "bill of rights," which is given to each patient at the time of admission.

Orders Not to Resuscitate is the result of a policy paper written with the help of physicians, lawyers, ethicists, and scholars, and was designed to provide a rational basis for decisions that the hospital staff routinely makes. An ad hoc committee of physicians and nurses responsible for the care of the patient, plus at least one other senior physician not involved in the case, focuses on whether the patient's death is so certain and so imminent that resuscitation would serve no purpose. Once this decision is made on physiological grounds, the responsibility for deciding whether to issue the orders not to resuscitate shifts to the patient (if he or she is competent) or to family members. Where there is no consent, there are no orders not to resuscitate. After an ONTR is issued, the patient's course is reviewed at least daily. If the patient's condition alters in such a way that survival is even remotely possible, the orders are revoked.

Although the Beth Israel approach deals only with resuscitation, not with the whole gamut of life-extending technologies that are often inflicted on dying patients, and is restricted to patients who are competent or have family members to give their consent (and is thus not pertinent to people like Walden Asbury), it is an important step in helping to clarify how the dying can die without being abused by technology. Orders not to resuscitate are not unique to Beth Israel. They are frequently written in medical charts. But what was once informal is now a codified procedure.

The Massachusetts General and Beth Israel approaches for humanely treating the dying hit a serious operational snag when the Massachusetts Supreme Judicial Court ruled, on November 28, 1977, that withholding and terminating critical care for any incompetent person — for example, a comatose or unconscious stroke victim or cancer patient, or a severely ill newborn — are matters for the probate courts to decide, not for families, doctors, nurses, social workers, priests, or committees. The ruling, in one swoop, could eliminate the procedural advances made by hospitals in trying to humanize death in a technological age.

*

In a system devised at the Los Angeles County–University of Southern California Medical Center, the dying patients themselves are the ones making the decision not to use any heroic measures. People burned beyond hope are asked whether they want doctors to try to keep them alive with last-ditch methods or let them die quietly.

For a few hours after their critical injury, it is believed that even badly burned patients feel little pain and can think clearly. A physician-nurse team, Bruce Zawacki and Sharon Imbus, seeking to recognize patient autonomy in decision-making, uses those few hours of lucidity to inform patients of their medical status, the available therapeutic alternatives, and their consequences. Survival for these patients is unprecedented, no matter what treatments have been used. The patients, armed with this information, may give — or withhold — permission to receive a particular form of treatment.

During a two-year period, of 108 adults who died in the burn unit, twenty-four were diagnosed on admission as having injuries without precedent of survival. Twenty-one of the patients or their families chose to have no heroic medical care. The three who chose full-treatment measures received them, but died anyway, as predicted.

Two sisters, sixty-eight and seventy years old, were in their car, waiting for a stoplight, when a nearby construction machine hit a gasoline line. The spraying gas exploded, leveled a city block, and ignited their car. The younger sister had burns over 92 percent of her body; the older one suffered burns over 95 percent of her body. Both were weakened from massive smoke inhalation.

The burn team agreed that survival was unprecedented in both cases, and discussed this with the sisters. The sixty-eight-year-old accepted the fact of her death honestly. "Well, I never dreamed that life would end like this, but since we all have to go some time, I'd like to go quietly and comfortably." Her older sister, meanwhile, doubted whether her injuries were as serious as reported. "I feel so good, wouldn't I be hurting horribly if I were doing to die?" she questioned. After a period of denial, she too agreed to go along with her sister's decision to have no heroic measures taken.

The sisters' beds were placed next to each other so that they could see and touch each other. They discussed funeral arrangements, and then, in the next breath, joked about the damage done to their hair. The younger woman died several hours later, and her sister succumbed the next day.

Giving autonomy about the final decisions in life to people with burns so severe that survival is unprecedented affects only a very small percentage of the dying. Yet the University of Southern California Medical Center approach is an attempt to share the decision-making about one of the most important aspects of life. Patients are not plunged into despair and greater pain by knowing the truth of their impending death, but instead become peaceful. They try to live out their lives to the end, saying things that are important to them, making plans and farewells. They are not hopeless, because they are in command of themselves and in control of their deaths.

Preparing for Death: Living Wills and Legislative Efforts

More than fear of death itself is the fear of lingering death — and the loss of power to affect what happens. Medical technology has the power to convert a dying person into a mechanically maintained object for days, months, or years, without anyone taking, or even having, the authority to make a decision to turn off all the equipment.

"We theoretically have the right to refuse treatment," said Sidney D. Rosoff, president of the Society of the Right to Die, "but this right is muted in practice by circumstances — possibly by our own incompetence as death approaches, or by our family's unwillingness or inability to support our wishes at that time."

Fear of being in this mechanically maintained state indefinitely has driven hundreds of thousands of Americans to sign Living Wills. These documents assert an individual's right to self-determination over his or her own body. "If the situation should arise in which there is no reasonable expectation of my recovery from physical or mental disability," reads the Living Will distributed by the Euthanasia Educational Council in New York City, "I request that I be allowed to die and not be kept alive by artificial means or 'heroic measures.'"

From 1969, when the Living Will was first published, through September 1975, when the Quinlan case first became news, the Euthanasia Educational Council distributed 750,-000 copies of it. By the end of 1977, nearly twice as many requests for the will were received from concerned people, presumably afraid of ending their days as Karen Ann Quinlan is doing.

The Living Will does not provide the umbrella protection that one and a half million Americans seek from it. The will, for example, relies on the kindness of the physicians to execute it, rather than on a legal requirement. Physicians may do less than a patient would have wished, or they may do more. Some people want a minimum of medication; others want drugs to alleviate suffering, even if the quantities of drugs required will hasten their death.

"When you are comatose, you are out of the ballgame," said lawyer George Annas, director of Boston University's Center for Law and Health Sciences. "The best you can do is write a Living Will and hope that your wishes are followed. If you don't come out of the coma, there is nothing you can do about it. And if you *do* come out, then you are grateful that they used the heroic measures."

The fuzzy writing of the Living Will clouds its ultimate effectiveness. It calls for "no heroic measures" when there is "no reasonable expectation of recovery." But what are heroic measures, and what kind of recovery is reasonable? A fifty-year-old father of two young children is in an automobile accident and is rushed to the emergency room of the nearest hospital for treatment. His back is broken, and he is bleeding profusely internally. Massive blood transfusions and a respirator to help him breathe get him past a medical crisis, which had brought him near death. He survives, but is paralyzed from the chest down.

Were those measures heroic? Is permanent paralysis a reasonable expectation of recovery? If he had signed a Living Will, what should the physicians have done?

When Sara Jean Watkins was twenty-one years old, she signed a Living Will. A few months later she had a routine gallbladder operation, and during surgery she vomited and aspirated her own vomitus. This freak accident left Sara Jean permanently unable to breathe independently. "Chances of her survival were very poor," her doctor related, "but there was one thing that might have changed her chances: an experimental lung machine.

"She opted to live." He pointed to her picture, which he keeps on the wall of his office — a picture of her hooked up to the lung machine. "And she opted for greater reliance on technology even though she had recently signed a Living Will, protesting the use of such technology. But then she was well, and now she was suddenly sick and dying — and ready to try anything. She died in spite of all the extraordinary efforts."

Sara Jean changed her mind, but that was just as much her right as was signing the will a few months before. The Living Will, like any will, is revocable. It does not impose death; it honors rights and seeks to make medical decisions easier.

*

"The Living Will is not a panacea," Sidney Rosoff said, "but it does represent patients' wishes so that they can influence the course of treatment during illness. While the will is not binding, you would expect that doctors would follow your wishes."

In theory, Rosoff is right: a nationwide poll conducted in 1976 by the American Medical Association showed that an overwhelming majority of physicians try to respect dying patients' wishes not to use extraordinary measures to prolong life. About 71 percent of the physicians responding to the AMA poll said they ask each patient about his or her wishes regarding medical care during a terminal illness, and as many as 95 percent of those inquiring try to adhere to the terminally ill patient's preferences about the nature and extent of care.

How these physicians act in fact remains unknown. One Texan wanted to sign a Living Will because "when Gabriel blows his horn, no S.O.B. is going to keep me from going." And Avery Weisman, professor of psychiatry at Harvard Medical School and a member of the Euthanasia Educational Council's Medical Advisory Committee, has never signed a Living Will because, he said, "I know some doctors whom I wouldn't want in charge of telling me the time of day, let alone the time to die."

How much protection is actually gained by the hundreds

of thousands of people who requested a Living Will so that they wouldn't spend their last days like Karen Ann Quinlan? According to the Euthanasia Educational Council, courts uniformly hold that administering medical treatment that a person does not want — assuming that person is mentally competent — constitutes assault and battery.

*

The Living Will is not legally binding everywhere, but almost every state has introduced legislation to legalize the right to die, and eight states have passed laws approving it.

California led the way when, on January 1, 1977, the Natural Death Act went into force. It was the first law that made a Living Will valid, giving people the legal right not to be hooked up to a respirator or kept alive by other artificial means when they are terminally ill and death is imminent. This precedent-setting law had many — some think too many — caveats. For the will to be valid, a person not only must have a terminal condition but must wait two weeks after receiving the terminal diagnosis to sign the directive. The will is valid only for five years, and then it must be re-executed. It also is invalid for a woman who becomes pregnant.

There are no provisions in the California law for penalizing physicians who ignore a patient's Living Will, but failure to follow a patient's expressed wishes will constitute "unprofessional conduct." Meanwhile, physicians are protected by the law when they pull the plug.

As part of his reason for signing the historic bill, Governor Edmund G. Brown, a former Roman Catholic seminarian, said, "Machines should serve humans rather than the reverse." But because it is so narrowly conceived, the bill may make things worse for patients and their families. The California Medical Association is concerned that personal arrangements between a physician and the family to stop heroic measures for an unconscious or incompetent relative who hasn't signed a Living Will could lead to a homicide prosecution. And perhaps physicians will now become deaf to requests by patients and families to let death come unless there is a written directive.

The California law gives no assurances to anyone who fears arriving comatose at the emergency room, or being maintained like Karen Ann Quinlan after an accident or stroke. And it would do nothing to protect the dying burned patients in the University of Southern California Medical Center.

Whatever its technical flaws, the California Natural Death Act was a vitally needed step forward in asserting patients' rights to reject unwanted medical care. Within a year after its passage, seven other states — Idaho, Arkansas, New Mexico, Nevada, Oregon, Texas, and North Carolina — enacted some version of a right-to-die legislation. None was as restrictive as California's.

*

More states are likely to pass right-to-die legislation, but the courts have the potential for giving less restrictive interpretations of the right to die. The Supreme Court of New Jersey established, in "In the Matter of Karen Ann Quinlan," March 31, 1976, that the privilege of choosing death and the right to privacy in certain circumstances takes precedence over the duty of the state to preserve human life.

The court concluded, "We have no hesitancy in deciding [that Karen should not be compelled] to endure the unendurable, only to vegetate a few measurable months with no realistic possibility of returning to any semblance of cognitive or sapient life."

If a competent, terminally ill patient, riddled by cancer and suffering great pain, asked not to be resuscitated, the court reasoned, that person could not be kept against his or her will on a respirator as a matter of right of privacy. So, too, Karen Ann Quinlan's right of privacy is being violated if she is forced to remain wed to the life-support apparatus.

Will the courts or the state legislatures be the major instrument for applying to death the concept of self-determination? Both have assumed aggressive roles and have achieved commendable results. No matter how the issue is resolved, two million people will still die each year. But when the right to die in peace without the inappropriate use of life-extending technologies is clearly established, the anguish of death can be diminished and the ambiguity of dying eliminated.

*

Death was once a taboo topic. It was not openly discussed; preparations for it by the healthy were rarely made; and the sick were left to die, out of sight, in hospitals and nursing homes.

The dying are no longer hidden in the back corridors of hospitals; some even emerge to die in the comfort of their homes. But though there is an acceptance of death, there is also a rebellion against inappropriate medical interventions standing in the way. The problem is not insoluble, and hospital standards, Living Wills, legislation, and court decisions represent just the beginning of solutions to the conflicts medical technology has imposed on the dying.

IV

ETHICS-KEEPING

Chapter 12

Choices for a New Medical Morality

THE LIST of possible medical encounters that pose moral problems throughout life is unending. There is no escape from them, but there is an emerging awareness that the issues exist and that we are not helpless in the face of them.

⟨Physicians are beginning to think about the moral dimensions of medical practice.

⟨Ethics think-tanks are playing the role of social consciousness–raisers by probing moral questions about medicine.

⟨Public accountability is emerging as an important force while legislatures, professional review boards, and health insurance companies join forces to control the spread of costly new medical advances before their effectiveness and safety are clearly known.

⟨And ultimately, each man, woman, and child has the right — indeed, the responsibility — to manage his or her health affairs throughout life, up to the moment of death.

None of these approaches will alone resolve the ethical dilemmas of medicine, but together they represent hope for a more rational basis for the decisions that must be made about them.

Everyday Practice, Everyday Ethics

At a Veterans' Administration hospital in Hines, Illinois, Dr. Robert Fruin has spent twenty-five years working with men suffering from spinal cord injuries. "The quality of life for these men is pretty severe," said Fruin, talking about some of his paraplegic and quadraplegic patients. "These critically injured and severely disabled patients frequently face moral dilemmas. The ethical issue for most of them is not one of treating or not treating, but of costs. Many of the 'quads' could go home and lead a better life than they can in the hospital, but who is going to pay the costs of the special equipment they need for eating, sleeping, and being transported in hydraulic-lift vans?

"My generation," continued the fifty-two-year-old internist, "was concerned with saving lives at all costs, but technology has changed all that. Costs for catastrophic injuries could be intolerable, but we know that these costs can vary, depending on how far we go in treating the men. Everyone is entitled to a decent level of care, but who makes the decision about what that decent level is? Having everything electronically operated makes a better quality of life for a quadraplegic, and helps for independent living, but it isn't essential for a person's physical health."

Family practitioner Tim Schmitt is also concerned about the ethical impacts of his practice in Wadena, Minnesota, where he works with a group of four other doctors in a county with a population under 14,000, where the income is below the national poverty level and where physicians are in great demand. Thirty-two-year-old Schmitt sees 250 patients a week, delivers one third of the 300 babies born in the county annually, and, as coroner, investigates the 150 unattended deaths that take place each year.

Practicing in a rural area — removed from many of the technological advances and life-saving devices that are omnipresent in large hospital centers — has caused some of Schmitt's ethical dilemmas. "We have to handle what *we* perceive we can do well," he said. "We have to be aware of the newest technology, and to recommend it when it is needed. For example, newborns with serious congenital problems are air-ambulanced to the hospital at the University of Minnesota or to Fargo, North Dakota.

"Women with high-risk pregnancies are also transferred to major hospital centers. Both the mother and child are our patients, and we have to grapple with human value issues for each one — weighing the naturalness of a delivery in a local setting against the mother and baby being thousands of miles away from home in a hospital center so that appropriate treatment can be given — *in case* a baby is born in trouble."

These are some of the concerns of two practicing physicians who are consciously seeking to incorporate an ethics perspective into their daily practice. There are thousands more like them — wanting to bring humanism into a traditionally scientific arena — but Robert Fruin and Tim Schmitt have done something about it. They exchanged one month of the hassle of clinical medicine for one month steeped in the study of medical ethics, values, and morals in a seminar program set up for medical professionals by the National Endowment for the Humanities (NEH). Others in the group included nurses, psychiatrists, a social worker, a genetics counselor, a hospital administrator, and a federal health-policy planner — all health-care professionals who wanted to explore current dilemmas in medical practice and health policy.

The impact of this blitz course, and five others like it sponsored by NEH at various teaching centers across the country, is not known. It affects only a small group of men and women, but nonetheless it is a start for concerned practitioners like Fruin, who received professional training in the dark ages of the 1940s and 1950s, "when science was the only thing that mattered in medical school."

*

"There is a great deal of confusion about what role the physician should play in making moral decisions," said Joseph Sheehan, chairman of the Department of Medical Education and Research at the University of Connecticut Health Center. "When a physician gives moral advice, it is equated — wrongly, as it turns out — with medical advice. But physicians have not been trained morally. Medical schools are intellectually stifling, and reflective reasoning is a luxury for medical students."

To help the next generation of doctors cope with the many ethical issues that will confront them during their years of practice, more and more medical schools are turning to formal courses in medical ethics. Through lectures, seminars, classes, workshops, and psychodramas, students probe the ethical dilemmas that surface in clinical practice — dilemmas that have developed because of technology's ability to blur some of the old distinctions between life and death, between benefit and risk, between helping and harming.

"Medical students should know more about the sick person's world if they are to care for sick people later on," says the Reverend David C. Duncombe, chaplain of the Yale Medical School. "And the best person to teach about the sick are the sick themselves."

Accordingly, each student in Duncombe's Seminar on the Chronically Ill is assigned to meet weekly with a patient whose life and social relationships are significantly compromised by a chronic, and in most cases, terminal illness. By interviewing patients, spending time with them, and getting to know them, students develop a sense of what it is like to live with a chronic disease and the constant threat of death. Death is so imminent for many of the patients that more than one third of them die during the semester. "This forces the student to get into an area that has a tremendous amount of meaning — death. It also gets them into emotional areas of medicine, which are then discussed in weekly class meetings," Duncombe explained.

Thrive as they may, medical ethics courses will not be able

to teach sensitivity, humaneness, and a system of morality, the way biochemistry can be taught. A physician who takes a medical ethics course will not necessarily become warm and sensitive. Rather, what medical ethics courses teach is more indirect — a gradual increase in awareness of different kinds of values and moral convictions. Deciding that a side effect is too great a risk, that relatives should be brought in for a consultation, or that medical records should or should not routinely be transmitted to patients — these are all decisions that rest on values, and should be recognized as the core of medical ethics issues.

Students and doctors alike have much to learn about medical ethics. They not only have to resolve some of the dilemmas for themselves; they have to be able to present difficult, ethically laden medical situations to patients and their families, who, after all, will ultimately decide what to do.

Ethical Watchdogs

A small band of ethics keepers is beginning to succeed in making biomedical researchers and practicing physicians aware of the ethical and societal significance of their work. The Hastings Center and the Joseph and Rose Kennedy Institute for the Study of Human Reproduction and Bioethics, the leading ethics think-tanks, are also influencing legislators and health-policy makers. Slowly — some think too slowly — they are raising social consciousness about medical issues.

"In the field of medicine and biology," said Daniel Callahan, of the Hastings Center, "many of our present decisions have implications for large numbers of people both living and yet to be born." Since 1969, the center, with its two dozen resident researchers and eighty-five fellows scattered in institutions around the country — a mixture of scientists and humanists — has been investigating some of these implications. More to the point, it has taken inherently ethical topics out of the ivory tower and brought them directly to the public.

After analyzing the moral implications of genetic screening,

Hastings researchers published guidelines in the *New England Journal of Medicine*, recommending that mass genetic screening be confidential, have back-up services and counseling, and that it be voluntary. This was at the time when many blacks had mandatory screening for sickle cell anemia. There was widespread misuse of the screening results, and virtually no follow-up for counseling. At least six states adopted the Hastings guidelines, and others modified their screening requirements.

Similarly, after long discussions on the definition of death, the center's staff developed a model code, which holds that a person shall be pronounced dead when the brain is destroyed — an ethical concept — but leaves to doctors the methods of reaching that determination. Nearly a dozen states have modified their statutory definition of death to conform in varying degrees to the center's model.

Half of the center's work is to crystallize thinking on bioethical issues through research activities in five major areas — death and dying, population, health policy, genetics, and behavior control. The other half is education — through the numerous books written by its researchers, the monthly *Hastings Center Report*, and workshops on the teaching of medical ethics.

The Kennedy Institute for the Study of Human Reproduction and Bioethics,* affiliated with Georgetown University in Washington, D.C., is a scholarly retreat for bioethicists. Since 1971, the institute has amassed the world's largest library specifically devoted to biomedical ethics. On its shelves are more than 4000 books, 11,000 catalogued articles, and scores of books written by the institute's resident scholars. LeRoy Walters, director of the institute's Center for Bioethics, edits the annual *Bibliography of Bioethics*, and a special staff was

---

* The Kennedy Institute is divided into three parts: the Center for Bioethics, the Center for Population Research, and the Laboratories for Reproductive Biology.

assembled to prepare the one-million-word *Encyclopedia of Bioethics*, which covers more than 350 topics written by leading scholars in ethics and medicine from around the world. The institute's scholars, an interdisciplinary team of physicians, philosophers, theologians, lawyers, and social scientists, explore a range of topics in bioethics and the philosophy of medicine, including research involving children and prisoners, humane treatment for the terminally ill, the just allocation of health-care resources, and the very definition of "health."

For research to be effective, however, it must reach a wider audience, and the Kennedy Institute scholars bring the results of their research to the public in a variety of ways. The data from the *Bibliography of Bioethics* are now made available to other researchers and students through the National Library of Medicine's computerized information network. Those actually working in the health field — physicians, nurses, health-care administrators and policy makers — are introduced to bioethics in an institute-sponsored one-week intensive course, and Washington health-policy makers attend monthly seminars on science, technology, and ethics. In perhaps their most forceful public effort, the institute scholars serve as members of various ethical review boards, including the Ethical Advisory Board of the Secretary of Health, Education, and Welfare, the Recombinant DNA Advisory Committee of the National Institutes of Health, Georgetown Medical School's Institutional Review Board, and the staff of the National Commission for the Protection of Human Subjects.

There are numerous other biomedical ethics centers — most of them affiliated with universities and medical schools — following the Kennedy Institute–Hastings Center models. And with due credit to them all, questions about biomedical ethics are no longer completely bypassed. They are being raised, and raised early enough so that legislators contemplating bills on the right to die, researchers working on recombinant DNA, and others in decision-making positions have time to consider them, and sometimes even to resolve them.

Public Accountability

The power behind technological control over life and death is too great to be left in the hands of a select group, and increasingly nonscientists are called on to help make decisions about health issues that were formerly left to scientists. Several states have nonphysicians on medical licensing boards, and a review board monitoring the incidence of adverse reactions to prescription drugs includes several public-interest lawyers and consumer advocates.

The use of lay members — public-interest lawyers, community and minority group representatives, clergy and ethicists — in decision-making positions in medical areas helps to ensure that decisions will not be made by scientific experts with vested interests. Senator Edward Kennedy proposed an eleven-member regulatory commission, with a majority of nonscientists, as a way to resolve the most emotionally laden biomedical debate of the 1970s — recombinant DNA. According to the Kennedy plan, none of the commissioners could have any past or present financial interest in DNA research. Scientists who want to do the controversial gene-splicing would have to apply for and receive a license from the commission, and agree to let commission-appointed investigators periodically inspect their laboratories to ensure adherence to the most stringent safety requirements. Kennedy withdrew support for his bill not because of disagreement over the role of the commission but because of the still unsettled dispute over the actual danger of DNA experiments.

The 1974 law that established the National Commission for the Protection of Human Subjects of Biomedical and Behavioral Research similarly calls for eleven members from a wide variety of specialty areas — the biological and physical sciences, theology, medicine, law, ethics, philosophy, health administration, and the social sciences. Not more than five of the commissioners can be people who are or were involved in biomedical or behavioral research involving human subjects. Clearly, the special knowledge acquired by biomedical researchers was necessary to help the commission investigate and make recommendations to the Secretary of HEW on such sensitive areas as practicing experimental medicine on fetuses, prisoners, children, and the mentally incompetent. But letting the majority vote lie in the hands of medical researchers — whose own research might be affected by an adverse vote — is no longer acceptable in today's biomedical ethical climate.

The message is clear: health-care policy and decisions are too important to be left to the medical experts. Medical decisions are seldom strictly medical, and they almost inevitably involve some judgments for which physicians have no special training or authority.

In 1965, the then-director of the National Institutes of Health, James A. Shannon, planted the seeds for broadening the mechanism by which medical research that involves human subjects is reviewed. Previously, collegial or peer approval was sufficient, but Shannon realized that "to win general acceptance within not only the medical research community but also our society at large, the final statement of [research] principles should probably emerge from a group which includes representatives of the whole ethical, moral and legal interests of society."

What subsequently emerged was a requirement that an institutional review board (IRB) must approve of the ethical merits of each research project involving human subjects in each hospital and medical center that receives HEW research funds. Without IRB approval, no research project will be considered as a recipient of federal funds. Since virtually every medical center relies on federal funding for research, the IRBs wield tremendous power in determining the ethical quality of medical research nationwide.

"It would be wonderful to think that every medical researcher approached work thoughtfully," said Dr. Robert Greenstein, chairman of the Committee on Human Experimentation at the University of Connecticut Health Center, "but the requirements for IRBs came about because the review process was haphazard and half-assessed. There is a need for researchers to be accountable to the public."

Institutional review boards are predominantly composed of scientists, in spite of Shannon's call for nonscientists as decision makers on medical research issues. But about thirty percent of the IRBs are composed of "others" — administrators, lawyers, nurses, clergy, ethicists, community representatives. The nonscientists tend to protect the research subject and place more emphasis on informed-consent procedures and on issues of privacy and confidentiality. The scientists, in contrast and not surprisingly, tend to balance the need for protecting the subject with the need to develop new medical knowledge.

IRBs have been criticized for trivializing the research process — by, for example, reviewing such riskless procedures as the collection of urine and blood. Another problem is that there are no specific guidelines for the operations of IRBs. Some meet in closed sessions; others are open to the public. Some review all procedures, even taking blood and urine samples; others have procedures for screening out proposals that do not need committee attention. Some have community representatives; others do not. Majority vote is required one place; unanimity in another. Each board is unique to the institution it represents. Would a review board in Boston agree with one in Des Moines? Would a committee with a Unitarian minister come to the same conclusions as one with a Southern Baptist minister or a Catholic priest? Is it necessary that all boards agree?

The IRB process cannot solve all the ethical problems in medical research. But it has brought many of the debates out of the laboratory and to the attention of the public, whose lives and welfare will benefit — or be at risk — as a result of the research.

He Who Pays the Piper Calls the Tune

Review boards and think-tanks, however helpful in raising consciousness and formulating guidelines, do not pay the bills.

In spite of the American dream of unlimited resources, the funds to save lives are not without bounds, and the time-honored medical view that a human life is priceless and that no cost should be spared to save it is now being criticized by health-care professionals.

("Most citizens pale at the specter of a city filled with non-agenarian stroke victims on tax-supported respirators, while garbage collection has ceased because of a lack of funds," wrote a physician in the *New England Journal of Medicine*. "If resources are indeed limited, some compromise between the actual performance and the enormous capabilities of medicine must be reached to avoid social bankruptcy."

("The money is there," commented a health-care analyst at Princeton, "but our priorities are wrong. Americans spend over twenty-two billion dollars on alcoholic beverages, four-teen billion on tobacco products, and some eighty billion on clothing and jewelry a year. If we have money for cigarettes and other frivolities, some less drastic trade-offs can be found before we deny someone the right to health or life."

(National priorities must be set to decide who should be helped and by what methods, concluded three medical professors who edited *Costs, Risks and Benefits of Surgery*. "We are developing life-saving methods well beyond our capacities to pay for them."

*

These are not isolated thoughts of doomsday critics; rather, they represent the ideas of a growing minority of the medical establishment who are concerned about the future of health care — about the ways in which we live and die.

The third-party payers — insurance companies and the federal Medicare and Medicaid programs — have a powerful role in determining national priorities for health-care spending because they decide what bills they will pay. They are beginning to show their clout by reimbursing for CAT scans only when the procedure is done on machines that have been approved with a certificate of need issued by an official state agency. And

the Blue Shield Association — insurers of medical costs for
seventy-two million people — has stopped routine payments
for twenty-eight questionable and generally discredited procedures, which were performed to the tune of over $25 million
annually for Blue Shield subscribers. The axed procedures —
most of them little-known operations on kidneys, uterus, nerve
and connective tissues, and arteries — were no longer effective
because new technologies had taken their place; they were
redundant when used with other procedures or could be repeated indefinitely without yielding any additional information. Thus, unnecessary procedures that were costly, risky,
and of questionable usefulness have been eliminated in one
clean sweep — not by ethics keepers but by bill-payers.

Each dollar of money directed toward medical research and
health care represents a value choice. "Policy-making," said
LeRoy Walters, of the Kennedy Institute, "always involves the
setting of priorities, and the priorities one chooses reflect the
values one wishes to maximize. Thus, there is always a significant ethical component in the policy-making process."

How much should the government spend on the delivery of
health-care services for today's patients? How much of the research should go for future generations? Should the government promote inexpensive intervention at an early stage of a
disease rather than costly last-ditch methods to alleviate some
of the damage? Each cost decision conceals a value decision.
The decision of policy makers to pay for hemodialysis, hip replacements, and other technical procedures for the aged, but
not for social care, counseling, or homemaker services, has a
major impact on the opportunities of the old to live independently.

If the government decides to pay for the blood-clotting factor for hemophiliacs, is it also obliged to pay for this costly resource for each subsequent hemophiliac born into the same
family? Should the government, in an effort to save money,
try to encourage parents to turn to other means in order not
to have additional hemophiliac children — adoption, foster
children, or abortion if a male is detected by amniocentesis,

since each male in a hemophiliac family has a fifty percent chance of having the disease?

Health-care priorities are beginning to be established as a means of cutting costs, but will the social and ethical implications be so restrictive and coercive that the benefits will not be worth it?

"The federal government is least equipped to say whether a medical service is ethical or moral," said Stanley Jones, a health-policy planner at the Institute of Medicine. "The government can't manage decisions in the abortion and pulling-the-plug category, because they are so value-laden at root."

Government involvement in medical decision-making has historically sought safer ground in providing health services, from free neighborhood clinics to fluoridation of water in more than half of the states, and in setting standards and regulations, such as permitting or banning a certain drug on the market, or requiring a certificate of need for expensive federally financed hospital equipment like CAT scanners. More expensive machinery and medical procedures, such as the coronary artery bypass, are likely to come under public scrutiny and review, not because of ethics or even concern for good medical care, but because of soaring and out-of-control medical costs.

Federal clout in health care, as in all areas of public spending, is most apparent in congressional appropriations. The 1977 abortion debate, which resulted in a decision to limit the use of federal funds for abortions, is a classic example of legislating ethics.

"Legislatures get carried away by what they feel is public opinion," said Angela Holder, counsel for medicolegal affairs at Yale–New Haven Hospital and former director of Yale's Law, Science, and Medicine Program. "The loudest-clamoring group gets the law. That is why the people with end-stage renal disease have federal reimbursement for their health care while the hemophiliacs don't.

"Basic constitutional rights, such as the right to life, should not be subject to popular vote. They are protected by the Bill of Rights, and should be fought for in the courts. Courts are more responsive in dealing with life-and-death issues. They can deal with the rule and the exceptions to it. Courts do not make uniform policy, but that should not be a deterring factor, because life isn't uniform."

Whether the courts or legislatures are more appropriate places for making bioethics decisions is moot, because the courts are doing it by default. Courts have run the gamut of bioethics decisions — from defining fetal viability in the Edelin case to allowing Karen Ann Quinlan's respirator to be disconnected.

*

One of the keys to resolving biomedical ethics issues in the future is prevention — eliminating the very need for medical encounters.

The average American man could have eleven additional years of life, and the average American woman, seven more years, if they exercised regularly, maintained moderate weight, ate breakfast and avoided snacks, didn't smoke, limited liquor consumption, and slept at least seven hours a night. Think of it — a longer and healthier life gained purely by common sense, and not a technological advance to thank.

The American love affair with medical technology persists, however, and it will continue until it is realized that more health services are not equated with longer and healthier lives.

The technological power to cure, treat, and prevent illness is a strong one, but even stronger is each individual's decision to use these medical advances rationally. This may be the biggest medical ethical choice of all.

NOTES
A Guide to Information
about Medical Choices

INDEX

Notes

CHAPTER 1 : Medical Mores   (*pages 1–15*)

The medical ethics issues about which George Bernard Shaw wrote in the 1911 appendix to *The Doctor's Dilemma* are startingly contemporary: the allocation of scarce resources, the popular desire to have the latest medical procedure performed whether or not it is efficacious or even safe, unnecessary surgery, and the presumed infallibility of physicians.

Picking up where Shaw left off, the *Encyclopedia of Bioethics* (Free Press, 1978) is an invaluable guide through the maze of medical dilemmas. The *Hastings Center Report,* a bimonthly publication of the Institute of Society, Ethics and the Life Sciences, in Hastings-on-Hudson, N.Y., analyzes current issues in medical ethics, from the right to be born to the right to die. The Hastings Center also publishes and updates each year a selected and partially annotated bibliography. The *Bibliography of Bioethics* (Gale Research Co.) is compiled annually by LeRoy Walters and is a part of the National Library of Medicine's computerized information network.

For in overview of the role of medical technology, I refer the reader to "Doing Better and Feeling Worse: Health in the United States," in the Winter 1977 issue of *Daedalus.* Lewis Thomas explains his theory of halfway technology there and in the *Bulletin of the American College of Surgeons,* June 1974, vol. 59, pp. 25–35. *Assessing Biomedical Technologies* (National Academy of Sciences, 1975) investigates potential advances and problems of *in vitro* fertilization, choosing sex of children, retarding the aging process, and modifying human behavior. *The Development of Medical Technology* (U.S. Congress, Office of Technology Assessment, August 1976) reviews nine medical technologies and the implications they present to society.

The Carter and Chambers cases were related to me by the patients' physicians; Annie Oliphant told me the story of her husband, Sloan; and Gail Kalmowitz's case was reported in the

New York Times, March 25, 1975. Dr. Bertrand Bell discussed public confidence in medicine in a personal interview, and the Mount Sinai (Chicago) survey was reported in *Medical World News*, February 2, 1977, p. 10.

An overview of medical ethics codes is available in the *Encyclopedia of Bioethics*. Daniel Callahan writes extensively on the definition of health in the *Hastings Center Report*, and Tristram Engelhardt's discussions on the philosophy of medicine are published frequently in the *Journal of Medicine and Philosophy*.

The issue of informed consent is discussed throughout *Experimentation with Human Subjects*, edited by Paul A. Freund (George Braziller, 1970). The Cleveland Clinic study was reported by Dr. Ralph J. Alfidi in the *Journal of the American Medical Association* (JAMA), May 24, 1971, vol. 216, pp. 1325–29. Further information about the Montifiore experience can be obtained from Dr. George Robinson, Albert Einstein College of Medicine, the Bronx, N.Y.

Chapter 2 : Creating a New Life   (*pages 19–41*)

The definition of life — or what constitutes viable life for a fetus — is discussed in *Research on the Fetus*, a report by the National Commission for the Protection of Human Subjects of Biomedical and Behavioral Research, U.S. Department of Health, Education, and Welfare, 1975.

Problems and advances of infertility were discussed in interviews with Drs. John Berryman, Jay Grodin, and Cecil Jacobson, and numerous articles on the subject have appeared in popular women's magazines.

The controversial issue of egg transfer was reported first in the Italian press. Albert Rosenfeld discusses this development in *The Second Genesis: The Coming Control of Life* (Vintage Books, 1975). Drs. Robert Edwards and Patrick Steptoe reported their work in *Lancet*, April 24, 1976, pp. 880–82. Leon Kass's comments on the procedure were published in the *New England Journal of Medicine* (NEJM), November 18, 1972, vol. 285, pp. 1174–79. The advertisement for a womb-for-hire appeared in the San Francisco *Chronicle*, April 15, 1975, and was subsequently reported by the Associated Press.

Two instructive books for the lay public on genetic diseases are *Know Your Genes*, by Aubrey Milunsky (Houghton Mifflin, 1977), and *Is My Baby All Right: A Guide to Birth Defects*, by Virginia Apgar and Joan Beck (Trident Press, 1972). The National Institute of General Medical Sciences at the National Institutes of Health, in Bethesda, Md. 20014, disseminates public information about genetic diseases and prenatal detection, as does the National Foundation–March of Dimes, Box 2000, White Plains, N.Y. 10602, and the National Genetics Foundation, 250 West 57 Street, New York, N.Y. 10019.

Dr. Roscoe O. Brady discussed the ethics of prenatal diagnosis of Fabry's and Gaucher's diseases with me. John C. Fletcher presents an overview of ethical implications of prenatal diagnosis in the *Encyclopedia of Bioethics*. He also reported on psychological problems involved in prenatal detection in "The Brink: The Parent-Child Bond in the Genetic Revolution," in *Theological Studies*, September 1972, vol. 33, pp. 457–85.

Both Kay Katz and Carolyn Sinclair related their children's cases to me in personal interviews, and the Giordanos' case was told to me by their pediatrician and genetic counselor.

CHAPTER 3: Manipulating the Gene Pool (*pages 42–64*)

The description of phenylketonuria (PKU), sickle cell, Tay-Sachs, and Huntington's disease, as well as a review of genetic screening issues, are in the Milunsky and Apgar-Beck books cited in the notes for Chapter 2. *Ethical, Social and Legal Dimensions of Screening for Human Genetic Disease* contains several relevant articles prepared by the Genetics Research Group of the Hastings Center (National Foundation–March of Dimes Birth Defects Original Articles Series, 1974, vol. 10). *Genetic Screening: Programs, Principles and Research* (National Academy of Sciences, 1975) examines current genetic screening practices. Gene Bylinsky discussed the subject in "What Science Can Do About Hereditary Diseases," *Fortune*, September 1974.

Dr. Neil Holtzman discussed with me many of the problems of mass screening for PKU, and he has published numerous articles on this in the *New England Journal of Medicine, the Journal of the American Medical Association,* and *Pediatrics.* Problems related to the PKU diet were explained by Elizabeth Walker and Sue Crosby, of the Maryland Department of Health. Ann Maguire gave testimony about her three PKU children at congressional hearings before the Subcommittee on Oversight and Investigations of the House Committee on Interstate and Foreign Commerce, "Shortchanging Children," October 7, 1975.

The National Foundation prepared an excellent historical review of sickle cell disease, and Philip Reilly reviewed genetic screening legislation in *Advances in Human Genetics,* vol. 5, 1975, pp. 319–69.

Details of the Tay-Sachs screening program are described in "Approaches to the Control and Prevention of Tay-Sachs Disease," by Michael M. Kaback, in *Progress in Medical Genetics,* vol. 10., 1974, pp. 103–34. The Montreal study of high school students is in *Pediatrics,* January 1977, vol. 59, pp. 86–91, and personal comments about the effects of Tay-Sachs screening were reported to me by genetic counselors.

Dr. Allen Crocker and John Fletcher discussed general issues of genetic counseling with me. Details of the couples interviewed by Fletcher were reported in his article, "The Brink," cited in the notes for Chapter 2.

The Commission for the Control of Huntington's Disease and Its Consequences, at the National Institutes of Health, Bethesda, Md. 20014, has accumulated significant data on the ethics of tests to detect presymptomatic victims. Nancy Wexler, executive director of the commission, interviewed several dozen families at risk for HD for her doctoral dissertation. Some of these families are quoted in this chapter.

April Murphy's case was reported by her physician, Dr. Mary G. Ampola, in the *New England Journal of Medicine,* August 14, 1975, vol. 293, pp. 313–17.

The controversial issue of using amniocentesis for sex-selection purposes was discussed by John Fletcher in his article on the ethics of prenatal detection in the *Encyclopedia of Bioethics.* He elaborated on this topic in a personal interview. The *Medical World News* survey is cited in a December 1, 1975, issue, in "Boy or Girl: Now Choice, Not Chance," by David Leff, pp. 45–56.

CHAPTER 4: Tomorrow's Genetics (*pages 65–80*)

The National Foundation–March of Dimes has published many accounts of the success story of David Camp; Larry Newell's story was reported in the Washington *Post*, November 30, 1975, in an article on hereditary cancer by Stuart Auerbach; April Murphy's case was cited in the notes for Chapter 3. All of these stories are exciting ones, but, as the chapter indicates, they pose dilemmas, some of which are described in "Ethical and Scientific Issues Posed by Human Uses of Molecular Genetics," *Annals of the New York Academy of Sciences*, vol. 265, January 1976.

Dr. Roscoe Brady's work on replacement therapy for Fabry's and Gaucher's diseases appears in the *New England Journal of Medicine*, July 5, 1973, vol. 289, pp. 9–14, and November 7, 1974, vol. 291, pp. 989–93. The case of the West German sisters was reported in *Medical World News*, August 25, 1975, p. 30.

The work of Carl Merrill was first reported in *Nature*, October 8, 1971, vol. 233, p. 370, and the artificial gene produced by a team headed by Har Gobind Khorana of MIT was reported widely in the popular press in the summer of 1976, when the news became public. Thomas H. Maugh II's article, "The Artificial Gene: It's Synthesized and It Works in Cells," *Science*, October 1, 1976, vol. 194, p. 44, explains Khorana's work clearly. Virtually every newspaper and magazine has had articles on recombinant DNA research, and several books have already been written on the topic, though the controversy is far from over. Nicholas Wade, a News and Comment writer for *Science* provides an excellent overview of the issue in *The Ultimate Experiment: Man-Made Evolution* (Walker and Co., 1977). *Science* provides in-depth coverage of recombinant DNA developments.

Genetic predispositions were described by Maya Pines in *Smithsonian*, July 1976, in "Genetic profiles will put our health in our own hands." *Genetics of Human Cancer*, a National Cancer Institute scientific volume edited by John Mulvhill, Robert Miller, and Joseph Fraumeni, Jr. (Raven Press, 1977), provides an explanation of the subject. Medicolegal aspects of familial cancer were raised by Patrick and Henry Lynch in the *Journal of Legal Medicine*, May 1976, pp. 10–16. The case of Karen McGinty and that of Theresa Boyd came from Lynch and from nurses

specializing in breast cancer. Drs. Fred Bergmann and Neil Holtzman expressed their concerns in personal interviews about the
implications of each person's genetic heritage being known.

"Heart Risk: Like Father, Like Son," appeared in *Medical
World News*, January 1, 1977, p. 89, and William A. Knaus reviews some of the controversies of cholesterol, diet, and heart
disease in the Outlook section, Washington *Post*, July 17, 1977.
Tabitha Powledge raised the question as to whether genetic
screening can prevent occupational disease in *New Scientist*, September 2, 1976, pp. 486–88.

CHAPTER 5: Muddled Medical Decisions (*pages 83–
99*)

Each month, the *Hastings Center Report* includes a case study
in bioethics — an actual clinical situation that poses ethical issues.
Cases are analyzed by leading health and bioethics professionals.
The dilemma of Allan Barnes — whether to have his recurrent
skin tumor treated by surgery or immunology — was reported in
the April 1975, issue, pp. 19–20. More than 100 of these cases
are collected in *Case Studies in Medical Ethics*, by Robert M.
Veatch (Harvard University Press, 1977).

The emotional issue of choosing one form of breast cancer
treatment over another is described in popular books and magazine articles. These are often personal accounts of women who
faced the dilemma when they were diagnosed as having breast
cancer. Hearings on the treatment of breast cancer, with testimony from cancer specialists, were held by the Subcommittee on
Health, Senate Committee on Labor and Public Welfare, May
4, 1976.

Gaby Lewis's story was related to me by her father. The Joint
Commission of Prescription Use, a coalition of public and private
groups in Washington, D.C., is collecting data on the use of
drugs and adverse reactions to them. *The Medicine Show*, written
by the editors of *Consumer Reports* (Consumers' Union, 1974),
is a practical guide to buying and using prescription drugs.

The issue of unnecessary surgery is described in *Costs, Risks
and Benefits of Surgery*, edited by Drs. Benjamin Barnes, John
Bunker, and Frederick Mosteller (Oxford University Press, 1977).

The book describes surgical abuses, including gastric freezing, hysterectomies, appendectomies, and the cost and efficacy of intensive care units. *The Cost and Quality of Health Care: Unnecessary Surgery* is a document prepared, in January 1976, by the House Committee on Interstate and Foreign Commerce, Subcommittee on Oversight and Investigations. The *Annals of Internal Medicine*, September 1974, vol. 81, pp. 289–93, contains a report on coronary care during the past thirty years. The British report on coronary care units versus home care appears in the *British Medical Journal*, April 17, 1976, pp. 925–29.

Albert Jonsen and the Reverend David Duncombe discussed problems of iatrogenicity with me in personal interviews, and Ivan Illich, in his *Medical Nemesis* (Pantheon Books, 1976) expounded the view that modern medicine has reached the state where it is a major threat to health.

A supplement to *Pediatrics*, April 1976, vol. 57, features a report on the history of oxygen therapy and retrolental fibroplasia, prepared by the American Academy of Pediatrics' Committee on the Fetus and Newborn. Data on diethylstilbestrol are inconclusive, but the Public Citizen Health Research Group in Washington, D.C., and the National Institute of Child Health and Human Development, Bethesda, Md., are sources of information. The stories of the DES mothers were published in the *New York Times*, June 17, 1976, in "Repercussions of a Drug," by Nadine Brozan. The dangers of hormone use for tall teen-agers were raised in "Controlling Height," by Angela Haines, the *New York Times* magazine, April 4, 1976. "Second Neoplasm — a complication of cancer chemotherapy," appeared in the *New England Journal of Medicine*, July 28, 1977, vol. 297, pp. 213–14, and "Compassion in Medicine," by Bernard Barber was published in *NEJM*, October 21, 1976, vol. 295, pp. 939–43.

CHAPTER 6: Birth Pangs   (*pages 100–123*)

Albert Haverkamp discussed the problems of fetal monitoring with me. His data on fetal monitoring appears in the *American Journal of Obstetrics and Gynecology*, June 1, 1976, vol. 125, pp. 310–17. The U.S. Congress, Office of Technology Assessment, Washington, D.C., has prepared an in-depth report of the efficacy and safety of medical technology, including an analysis of fetal monitoring.

The most inclusive report on survival of very small babies was prepared by Drs. Richard E. Behrman and Tove S. Rosen, for the National Commission on the Protection of Human Subjects of Biomedical and Behavioral Research. Their report on viability and nonviability of the fetus is in the appendix of the commission's 1975 report, *Research on the Fetus*. The Los Angeles Cedars–Sinai Medical Center item on the costs of neonatal intensive care units was reported in *Medical World News*, October 3, 1977, p. 15.

The National Foundation–March of Dimes' two-day seminar on new directions in perinatal care, held in New York City, March 1977, included discussions on the effect of steroids on mature fetal lungs. Ethical considerations of steroid treatments are raised by Drs. Mary Ellen Avery and Victor Chernick in "On decision making surrounding drug therapy," the *New England Journal of Medicine*, January 13, 1977, vol. 296, pp. 102–103.

The cases of Linda Culbertson and Rosemarie Maniscalo were reported in the popular press at the time of the events — in November 1976 for Mrs. Culbertson and a year later for Mrs. Maniscalo. Laurie Goforth's case was reported in *Medical World News*, March 6, 1978, p. 14.

"Moral and Ethical Dilemmas in the Special-Care Nursery," by Drs. Raymond Duff and A. G. M. Campbell, appeared in the *New England Journal of Medicine*, October 25, 1973, vol. 289, pp. 890–94. *The Ethics of Newborn Intensive Care*, edited by Albert Jonsen and Michael Garland (University of California School of Medicine, San Francisco, and the Institute of Governmental Studies, Berkeley, 1976), provides an excellent overview of critical issues in treating very sick newborns.

The survey by the University of California School of Public Health at Berkeley on treating babies with Down's syndrome was reported in the *Hastings Center Report*, April 1976, p. 2. John Lorber's original article calling for criteria for treatment of spina bifida children appeared in *Developmental Medicine and Child Neurology*, 1971, vol. 13, pp. 279–303. An overview of ethical problems in the management of children with spina bifida was discussed in a two-part series Lorber wrote in *Nursing Times*, vol. 72, February 26 and March 25, 1976. Drs. Sherman S. Stein,

Luis Schut, and Mary Ames, of the Children's Center in Philadelphia, reported their selection criteria in *Pediatrics*, November
1974, vol. 54, pp. 553–57.

The personal cases in this chapter were related to me directly
by the families involved — the Barrs, LaFontaines, Holtons, and
Browns. Drs. Mary Kate Davitt, John Berryman, Raymond Duff,
and David McCullough, and nurse Catherine Quinn provided
much of the material and insights into problems in the neonatal
intensive care unit.

CHAPTER 7: Tools for Diagnosing   (*pages 124–142*)

Shoshanna Abeles and Gay Kroeger related to me, in personal
interviews, their experiences with the CAT scanner, and H. David
Banta, David Davis, and William Knaus briefed me on technological, economic, and ethics aspects of the scanner. Michael
Halloran's case and data on the St. Elizabeth's Home are cited in
"The Miracle Machine," by Judi Kesselman and Franklynn Peter-
son, in *Family Health/Today's Health*, January 1977. A review
of the spectacular popularity of the CAT scanner, *Health Policy
and the Computerized Tomograph Scanner*, was prepared by the
U.S. Congress, Office of Technology Assessment, Washington,
D.C.; and the Institute of Medicine issued a policy statement, *Computed Tomographic Scanning* (National Academy of
Sciences, April 1977). Drs. Stuart Shapiro and Stanley Wyman's
article, "CAT Fever," was printed in the *New England Journal of
Medicine*, April 22, 1976, vol. 294, pp. 954–56. Drs. Herbert
Abrams and Barbara McNeil reported on the medical implications of CAT scanning in *NEJM*, February 2 and February 9,
1978, vol. 298. Eliot Marshall discussed scanning in the *New Republic*, April 16, 1977, pp. 11–15, as part of a series on the
anatomy of health-care costs.

The National Cancer Institute, Bethesda, Md. 20014, prepared
a briefing document on the development of the breast cancer detection program. The personal experiences concerning mammography were related directly to me by the women involved or by
the health professionals who were caring for them. The risks in
transferring medical technology too rapidly were discussed in
"Breast Cancer Screening: A view from outside the controversy,"

by Dr. Samuel Thier, in the *New England Journal of Medicine*, November 10, 1977, vol. 297, pp. 1063–65. John Bailar III talked with me about the risks of mammography for women of all ages, and reported on the subject in "Mammography — A Time for Caution" in the *Journal of the American Medical Association*, March 7, 1977, vol. 237, pp. 997–98.

"Evaluating the Physician and His Technology," by Walsh McDermott, *Daedalus*, Winter 1977, is a discussion of some of the problems of diagnostic technologies, and "X-Rays: How Much is Too Much?", in *Medical World News*, December 27, 1976, pp. 30–40, raised current and historical questions about the safety of x-rays. The National Cancer Institute has prepared information for physicians as well as the general public on irradiation-related thyroid cancer. Priscilla W. Laws's data come from her report, *Medical and Dental X-Rays: A consumer's guide to avoiding unnecessary radiation exposure* (Public Citizen Health Research Group, 1974) and *X-Rays: More Harm Than Good* (Rodale Press, 1977).

"The Case Against Regular Physicals," by Richard Spark, appeared in the *New York Times* magazine, May 25, 1976. Walter McQuade stated his position in "Those Annual Physicals Are Worth the Trouble," in *Fortune*, January 1977. The systolic click syndrome was discussed in personal interviews with Drs. Michael Halberstam and Joseph Romeo, and the responses of four cardiologists to the question of the significance of systolic click appeared in *Modern Medicine*, October 15, 1976, pp. 56–61.

CHAPTER 8: The Body Shop   *(pages 143–163)*

For a provocative introduction to the problem of allocation of scarce resources, see James Childress's "Who Shall Live When Not All Can Live?", *Soundings*, Winter 1970, vol. 53, pp. 339–62, reprinted in *Readings on Ethical and Social Issues in Biomedicine*, edited by Richard W. Wertz (Prentice-Hall, 1973); and Henry Beecher's "Scarce Resources and Medical Advancement," in *Experimentation with Human Subjects*, edited by Paul A. Freund (George Braziller, 1970). Two excellent sources in dialysis and kidney transplants are *Catastrophic Diseases: Who Decides What?* by Jay Katz and Alexander Capron (Russell Sage

Foundation, 1975), and *The Courage to Fail: A Social View of Organ Transplants and Dialysis*, by Renée C. Fox and Judith P. Swazey (University of Chicago Press, 1974).

Lee Foster's account of his life on dialysis is recounted in the *Hastings Center Report*, June 1976, and *Reader's Digest*, September 1976. The case of the New York citizen who received a Russian kidney was reported in the *New York Times*, February 24, 1977. The rest of the personal data about end-stage renal disease come from interviews with physicians and patients at the Washington Hospital Center and at Georgetown University Hospital.

Shana Alexander's article, "They Decide Who Lives, Who Dies," *Life*, November 9, 1962, pp. 102–123, is the source of information about the Seattle God Committee. Richard Rettig, of the RAND Corporation, Washington, D.C., has written several policy papers on the federal kidney treatment program, including "Lessons Learned from the End-Stage Renal Disease Experience," November 1976. Eliot Marshal's "Rendezvous with a Machine," in the *New Republic*, March 19, 1977, pp. 16–19, is part of his anatomy of health-care costs series. Current data on the size and costs of the End-Stage Renal Disease Program are available from the Social Security Administration, Department of Health, Education, and Welfare, Baltimore, Md. 21235.

The Office of Science and Health Reports, Division of Research Reports, National Institutes of Health, Bethesda, Md., published Research Advances in Human Transplants, and Dr. Willard Gaylin wrote a provocative article, "Harvesting the Dead," published in *Harper's*, September 1974, pp. 23–27.

The debate over coronary artery bypass is reported on frequently in the *New England Journal of Medicine*. Among the articles is one on the Veterans' Administration study, September 22, 1977, vol. 297, pp. 621–26; an editorial on the lessons of the coronary artery bypass debate and a series of reader responses are in December 29, 1977, vol. 297, pp. 1462–70.

Heart transplants as a way of treating diseased and damaged hearts are discussed in the Katz-Capron book; and legal, social, ethical, medical, economic, and psychological implications of the totally implantable artificial heart are presented in a report of the Artificial Heart Assessment panel, National Heart and Lung Institute, Bethesda, Md., September 1973. The ethics committee of the American Heart Association published "Ethical Considerations of the Left Ventricular Assist Device," in the *Journal of the American Medical Association,* February 23, 1976, vol. 235, pp. 823–24.

Disease by Disease Toward National Health Insurance was published by the Institute of Medicine (National Academy of Sciences, 1973). Dr. James Hunt's remarks were quoted in "Kidney Program: A monstrosity?", in *Medical World News,* August 23, 1976. p. 37.

CHAPTER 9: Postponing Death   (*pages 167–188*)

Death, Dying and the Biological Revolution: Our Last Quest for Responsibility, by Robert M. Veatch (Yale University Press, 1976), presents an overview of the medical, ethical, and legal aspects of death and dying. New technologies that are being developed to extend life by increasing age span are discussed in *Prolongevity,* by Albert Rosenfeld (Alfred A. Knopf, 1976).

Conrad Taeuber discussed "If Nobody Died of Cancer . . . ?", in *Death and Dying: An examination of legislative and policy* issues. His article was a report given at a conference held on June 30, 1976, Washington, D.C., by the Health Policy Center, at Georgetown University, and the American Association for the Advancement of Science. Stanley Joel Reiser wrote about the papal statement in "Therapeutic Choice and Moral Doubt in a Technological Age," in *Daedalus,* Winter 1977. The Harvard Medical School Ad Hoc Committee to Examine the Definition of Brain Death published its findings in *Journal of the American Medical Association,* August 5, 1968, vol. 205, pp. 337–40. The observation of brain waves from a bowl of Jell-O was reported in the *New York Times,* March 6, 1976. Karen Ann Quinlan's case was reported extensively and somewhat sensationally in the popular press (see Joseph Healey's "The Quinlan Case and the Mass Media," in the *American Journal of Public Health,* March 1976, vol. 66, pp. 295–96). *In the Matter of Karen Ann Quinlan: The Complete Legal Briefs, Court Proceedings and Decision in the Superior Court of New Jersey* was published in 1975 (University Publications of America).

The cases of Stanley Wilks and Rodney Waldman were related

directly to me by family members and by physicians in charge of their care. Herman Feifel's "Who's Afraid of Death?" appeared in the *Journal of Abnormal Psychology*, 1973, vol. 81, pp. 282–88. Diana Crane also discussed physicians' reactions to death in her excellent book, *The Sanctity of Social Life: Physicians' Treatment of Critically Ill Patients* (Russell Sage Foundation, 1975).

The successful use of anticancer drugs is reported in Jane Brody and Arthur Holleb's *You Can Fight Cancer and Win* (Quadrangle, 1977). The side effects of chemotherapy are documented widely in medical journals; see *Cancer*, July 1975 supplement, vol. 36, "Successes in Cancer Treatment," "Prospectus for Cancer Treatment," and other papers presented at the Georgetown University Medical Center Cancer Symposium, Washington, D.C., January 18, 1974.

The cases of Edna Luzzata and Victor Billington were told to me by their physicians; Hubert Humphrey's story was widely reported in the press; Morris Abram's fight against cancer was told in the *New York Times*, August 15, 1977; and Danny Carter's attempt to extend his life with Laetrile was related to me by his family.

The *FDA Consumer*, a publication of the Food and Drug Administration, published "Laetrile: The Making of a Myth," December 1976–January 1977, and "Cancer Quackery: Past and Present," July–August 1977. A case study in bioethics from the *Hastings Center Report*, December 1976, pp. 18–20, is concerned with the ethics of whether patients should have access to an unapproved drug, and *Newsweek*, June 27, 1977, featured a cover story, "Laetrile: Should it be banned?" The case of the restaurant owner is cited in the *Newsweek* article, and the schoolteacher's story is in *Healing: A Doctor in Search of a Miracle*, by William A. Nolen (Random House, 1974).

Chapter 10: Deciding to Die   (*pages 189–208*)

This chapter is based on the personal stories of people who made the final decisions in their lives. The Brown case is cited in "Family Decision: A crucial factor in terminating life," by Jerry J. Griffin, in the *American Journal of Nursing*, May 1975, vol. 75, pp. 795–96. The Phillips case is discussed by a panel of physicians and nurses in Chapter 14 of "The Doctor Lets the Patient Die," in *Critical Incidents in Nursing,* edited by Loretta S. Bermosk and Raymond J. Corsini (W. B. Saunders, 1973). Senator Philip Hart's experience of dying at home was reported in the Washington *Star,* December 5, 1976.

The cases of Gabriel Oleaga and Sondra Sutter were described to me by their physicians; and the cases of Fern Terry, Samantha Teague, Jeffrey Sinclair, John Schuler were related by their parents, widows, and widowers. I viewed videotapes made by Richard Green and visited Mary Willis just before her death, while making home-care visits with Dr. Peter Petrucci and nurse Alise Green.

I also visited St. Christopher's Hospice, in London, and spoke with Dr. Cicely Saunders about the hospice approach to treating the dying. For further information about hospices in the United States, contact Hospice Action, P.O. Box 32331, Washington, D.C. 20007, and Hospice, Inc., 765 Prospect Street, New Haven, Conn. 06511.

CHAPTER 11: Pulling the Plug   (*pages 209–226*)

The cases of Watkins, Lipschultz, and Asbury were related to me by physicians on a surgical and burn intensive care unit in a major teaching hospital. They requested that they and the hospital remain anonymous.

The guidelines at Mount Sinai Hospital, New York, were first described by Garth Tagge, Christopher Bryan-Brown, and Diane Adler in *Critical Care Medicine,* 1974, vol. 2, pp. 61–63. Dr. Bryan-Brown discussed these categories in greater detail in a personal interview.

Dr. Ned Cassem spoke to the National Institutes of Health Ethics Seminar about the Massachusetts General Hospital's Critical Care and Optimum Care Committees. A report on these committees appears in the *New England Journal of Medicine,* August 12, 1976, vol. 295, pp. 362–64. Dr. Mitchell Rabkin discussed with me the development of Orders Not to Resuscitate at Beth Israel Hospital, and he wrote about them in the *New England Journal of Medicine,* August 12, 1976, vol. 295, pp. 364–66. "Autonomy for Burned Patients When Survival Is Unprecedented," by Sharon Imbus and Bruce Zawacki, appeared in the *New England Journal of Medicine*, August 11, 1977, vol. 297, pp. 308–310. Robert Veatch wrote "Hospital Ethics Committees: Is there a role?" in the *Hastings Center Report*, June 1977. In addition, the center held a conference on hospital ethics committees in April 1977. Diana Crane discussed the need for guidelines for the terminally ill in her book, *A Sanctity of Social Life*, cited in the notes for Chapter 9.

Sidney Rosoff and George Annas discussed with me some of the problems concerning Living Wills. Further information about the Living Will is available from the Euthanasia Educational Council, 250 West 57 Street, New York, N.Y. 10019. Sara Jean Watkins's case was told to me by the attending physician in an intensive care unit. A historical review of right-to-die efforts was presented by Sidney Rosoff at the Health Policy Center–American Association for the Advancement of Science conference and published in the proceedings, *Death and Dying*, cited in the notes for Chapter 9. Citations for the Quinlan case are also cited in Chapter 9. The Hastings Center published an analysis of legislative proposals on euthanasia and treatment refusal in November 1977, and an annual legislative manual is prepared by the Society for the Right to Die and is available through the Euthanasia Educational Council.

CHAPTER 12 : Choices for a New Medical Morality   (*pages 229–242*)

Drs. Robert Fruin and Tom Schmitt were interviewed while they were in Washington for the National Endowment for the Humanities Seminars for Medical Practitioners. Joseph Sheehan, at the University of Connecticut Health Center, and the Reverend David Duncombe, at Yale Medical School, described to me the teaching of medical ethics at their schools. Descriptions of other medical schools' ethics courses are in *Human Values Teaching Programs for Health Professionals* (Society for Health and Human Value, Philadelphia, 1976).

For information on the ethics think-tanks described in this chapter, write to the Hastings Center (The Institute of Society, Ethics and the Life Sciences), 360 Broadway, Hastings-on-Hudson, N.Y. 10706; and the Kennedy Institute for the Study of Human Reproduction and Bioethics, Georgetown University, Washington, D.C. 20057.

The National Commission for the Protection of Human Subjects of Biomedical and Behavioral Research, Westwood Building, 5333 Westbard Ave., Bethesda, Md. 20016, has copies, available to the public, of recommendations and reports on medical research on fetuses, prisoners, the mentally infirm, and children. They also commissioned numerous reports relevant to the biomedical research process, including a survey on the efficacy of institutional review boards and analyses of ethical principles in research and clinical practice.

The ethics and economics of health care are discussed by Victor R. Fuchs in *Who Shall Live: Health Economics and Social Choice* (Basic Books, 1974). Howard Hiatt raised questions of the future of health care in "Protecting the Medical Commons: Who is responsible?", in the *New England Journal of Medicine*, July 31, 1975, vol. 293, pp. 235–41. *Costs, Risks and Benefits of Surgery*, edited by Drs. Barnes, Bunker, and Mosteller, cited in the notes for Chapter 5, also contains much relevant data on the past, present, and future of the ethics and economics of health care. *The Complex Puzzle of Rising Health Care Costs: Can the private sector fit it together?* is a compendium of labor-management innovations in reducing health-care costs (Council on Wage and Price Stability, Executive Office of the President, Washington, D.C., December 1976). Details about third-party reimbursement policies are available from the headquarters of Blue Cross, Blue Shield, Aetna, etc. The Institute of Medicine policy statement about reimbursement for CAT scans is cited in the notes for Chapter 7. Angela Holder, Stanley Jones, and LeRoy Walters discussed their views of public policy and health care in personal interviews.

Index